Living With
Epidermolysis Bullosa

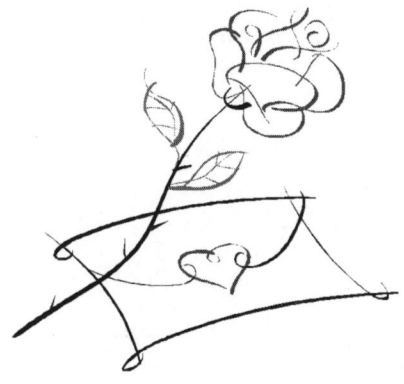

Compiled By

Silvia Corradin

Edited By

Brenda Gionfriddo

First Printing: 2007

ISBN: 978-1-4303-2886-5

Silvia Corradin
Lancaster, CA 93535

www.ebinfoworld.com

Table of Contents

Living with Epidermolysis Bullosa

Introduction

Epidermolysis Bullosa, EB. I never heard these words before, or had any knowledge this disorder existed until my son Nicholas was diagnosed with it about 12 hours after his birth on November 25th, 1996. A month later his official diagnosis came back as a "classic" case of Recessive Dystrophic.

While it was a devastating diagnose, at the time I was just happy to have a baby to hold, love and care for, as a mere 21 months earlier I had a baby that was stillborn at full term, Alex, and EB was now given to me as most likely the cause for his demise. The truth is, however, that back then I really had no understanding how devastating EB is, and, can be, and over the years I had a hard time explaining to friends and family what I was going through and that I was not exaggerating. It was only after some of them saw pictures or read my story that they understood, some even apologized. Perhaps this book will help families explain to their families and friends what they are going through as well.

As I write this, Nicky is 10.5 years old, and his health has its ups and downs, sometimes his wounds account to only 30% of his body, other times much more. These are second-degree burn-like wounds that are deep and take anywhere from a week to months and months to heal, some are as large as my fist or larger. His body needs to be covered in bandages to protect his healthy skin and allow his wounds to heal properly. Because his feet are so fragile, Nicky has a power chair to ease his walking.

Nicky also has a g-tube that supplies nutrition to him, as his mouth is too sore to eat anything that needs to be chewed or has a harsh texture. His tongue is fused to the bottom of his mouth and he has no gum space, as that's all fused together. He has had many throat dilatations, a few hand surgeries, countless blood transfusions and too many other problems to list. Skin is, after all, the largest organ we have, and it affects everything.

Despite it all, Nicky is my light and inspiration. He can be crying and upset about a wound one moment, and light up a room the next. Every teacher and Aide that he's had can't stop gushing on how much they love him, how funny he is and how amazing he is doing in school. Yeah… that's my guy! Nicky and I have so much fun together at times, he can be so funny, he's my little comedian, and while life has dealt him a major blow one can't help but know he has a Happy Heart. My story- and his- is the very last one in the book.

What is EB?

Epidermolysis Bullosa, EB, is a rare genetic skin disorder. One way to describe its rareness is that a doctor or a nurse can work a lifetime and never bump into this condition. It is estimated that about 10,000 Americans, mostly kids, have some form of EB. According to the latest United States figures, most of these patients suffer from the Simplex form of EB, about 600 have the Junctional form, 600 have RDEB, 840 with DDEB and 320 with some unclassified form of EB.

In simple terms, people born with EB lack anchors that hold the layers of their skin together. As a consequence, any activity that rubs or causes pressure produces a painful sore akin to a burn. One form of EB is lethal in the first weeks or months of life. Some are mutilating over time. Infection is a serious, ongoing concern. As if the diagnosis is not heartbreaking enough, no treatment for EB has been effective. Parents have coped by protecting the child's skin with gauze and ointments to prevent and protect the wounds and healthy skin-something that HMO's refuse to pay for.

The first reported cases of blistering diseases that would fall into the EB umbrella were initially noted in the late 1800, starting from about 1870. It wasn't until 1908 that at least one major dermatology textbook published in English used the term "Epidermolysis Bullosa" to describe patients with congenital blistering. Because the term was coined before the major differences between the subtypes were recorded and studied, while there are three forms of EB, they are widely different from one another.

The three main types of EB are Simplex, Junctional, and Dystrophic. The severity varies widely, with only a handful of true subtypes. The Simplex and "Dominant" Dystrophic are Dominant   forms, meaning that either the parent has the condition and has a 50% chance of passing it on to their child, or it's a fluke at conception. Normally these forms do improve with age for the most part. The other forms, Junctional and

"Recessive" Dystrophic, are all recessively inherited and are also more severe and lethal in most cases, as both parents need to be 'healthy' carriers, hence have a recessive gene for EB in their DNA. Two parents that are both carriers have a 25% chance of having a child with EB in each pregnancy.

This book has first-hand accounts written by parents and patients who are living or have lived with EB, and was compiled to help people in general understand how it is like to truly live with every form of Epidermolysis Bullosa, from the milder Simplex variants, who are nonetheless not simple to live with, to the more lethal, namely Junctional, whose patients usually succumb to before their first birthday. The stories you will read are from proud parents, or patients and their struggles and how they are coping. Some stories are sad, some are encouraging, and everything in between. I am hoping that it will also contain something useful for new parents of a baby with EB, and for those who would just like to know they are not alone or anyone who simply wishes to learn more about EB.

The information in this book isn't exhaustive, and it isn't intended to replace discussions with your doctor or any other professional. But it should provide an introduction to the key issues involved in living with EB.

I would like to take a moment and thank all the families that took time out of their busy daily life to submit their stories for this book. For more information about EB, please visit my website at: http://www.ebinfoworld.com

Please refer to the back of the book for a complete listing of all EB organizations that help EB families worldwide.

Many Blessings
Silvia Corradin
June 3, 2007

Living with Epidermolysis Bullosa

Life Stories

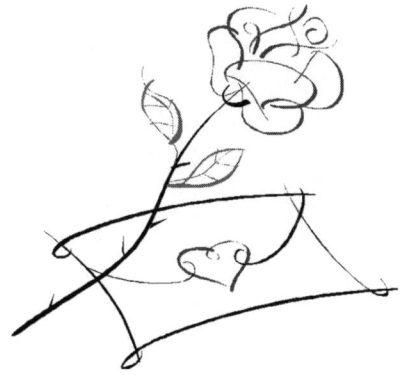

When we long for life without difficulties,
Remind us that oaks grow strong in contrary winds
And diamonds are made under pressure.

- Peter Marshall

Living with Epidermolysis Bullosa

Tomorrow's Promise?

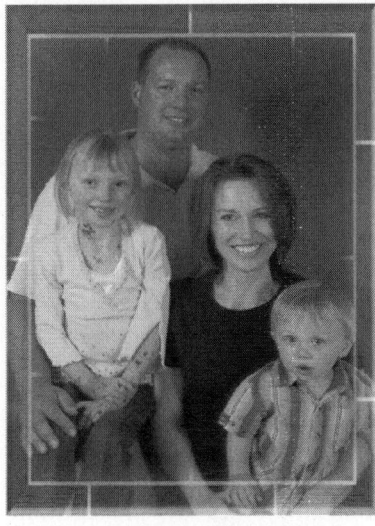

By Doug & Terry S.
Wisconsin, USA

Doug and Terri S. are the parents of Faith, a 6.5 year old girl with Junctional Epidermolysis Bullosa. After years of testing they were able to have a boy without Faith's complications. This is a view into a day in the life of Faith.

You hear the voices from the morning news in the background as a blonde haired little boy is clinging to his mother in the kitchen to exhaust every last bit of attention and love he can get from her as if he has been starved of affection since his birth just 18 months earlier. There is a beagle named Jack still asleep on his cushion that was placed in the corner of his owner's bedroom where he is supposed to be in the morning, yet most mornings you can find him curled up in the big comfy chair that is strictly off limits to a dog, unless he is sneaky enough to make his way out to the chair in the middle of the night. It seems the scolding he gets when caught in the morning by his owner on the way out the door to work is starting to pay off.

At the end of a long hallway covered in family photos, you can still catch a glimpse of the night-light shining from a room that has not yet been drowned out by the morning sun. It is in this room that sleeps an extraordinary little girl. This little girl called Faith, by just simply meeting her, can make you feel like the luckiest person in the world, the most selfish person in the world, the most humble person in the world. This list could go on for quite some time so let me explain what I mean.

Faith's affliction is a disease called Epidermolysis Bullosa, which she was diagnosed with at birth. This disease causes her skin to blister from the slightest friction, and unlike a blister that people without this affliction would get; they need to be popped as quickly as they are discovered as not to allow them to grow larger and larger.
As you might think an active little girl only six years old can accumulate a number of blisters and sores all over her body, making them readily visible to the casual observer.

Her mom calls from the kitchen; time to get up sweetie you need to get ready for school. A few minutes pass when Terri realizes she's going to have to make an appearance to motivate Faith from her nest. As Terri makes the turn to the room, Cal who knows it's time to wake his favorite playmate up passes her. Terri can already see the curves of a grin made by her thinking she has just pulled one over on her mom.

This is just one of the games Faith likes to play, to see how worked up she can get her little brother and make sure she is welcomed into the new day by her mom.

The bloodstains on the pillowcases from the sores on her face would make most people think that Faith had a hard night of sleep but the smile on her face tells her mom otherwise. She gets out of bed and none of the sores have dried and stuck to the sheets, two for two, the morning is looking good.

Faith walks to the bathroom gingerly on her feet with a little wince of pain in every step but doesn't let on that there is any cause for concern as she does every morning.

Terri asks what she would like for breakfast. Faith wants the leftover pancakes her dad made on Sunday morning that she likes so much, not because she likes pancakes particularly but she likes the times when everyone is together at once, but it's already Tuesday and they have been eaten, so she picks the next best thing for a six year old, Lucky Charms. Faith prolongs breakfast to the point if she could tie it in with lunch she would, because she knows after breakfast she needs to get dressed for school and that means popping any blisters and changing dressings on sores that occurred overnight.

You can see it in her face she wishes she could go to some far off place in her mind as if it wasn't really happening and sometimes it seems you can see it in her eyes, she is actually there and numb to the needle that pierces the blister and the bandages that cover the sores. But when the needle catches a nerve or the bandages need to be replaced it becomes all too much a reality again.

The bandages will stick to the open sores and when replaced they are rubbed with a petroleum jelly and antibiotic blend to help loosen the bandages from the wounds. Sometimes this seems more like a placebo to help Faith with the pain, she knows is on the other side of the bandage.

Today was not bad, some blisters on the hand that are about the size of eraser tips needed to pierced and drained but her back and elbows look good and the sores on her bottom have healed nicely. When Faith is in her underwear waiting for her mom to put her clothes on, you can see red blemishes against her pale skin of blisters that have come and gone but left a glimpse of how fragile she is and how quickly they are willing to return if disturbed. On her birdlike legs you can see the shiny almost tissue paper like skin on her shins and knees. The skin that covers muscular or soft tissue areas takes on a much different look then areas that don't.

Faith is dressed in her favorite color of pink and now that this part of her day is over, the transformation into an energetic kid excited for school and the opportunity to play with her friends shines through. To this day, it is an enigma how quickly she can block out what most people would consider a traumatic experience and move forward through the day with a smile on her face.

Cal is doing his self-appointed job of bringing everyone his or her shoes, because taking Faith to school is a new adventure he looks forward to everyday.

Faith thanks her brother for the kind gesture and gives him a hug as he looks on with a grin so large as if he just found the cure for his sister's daily regimen, that he has witnessed everyday of his short life. I can't help but be curious how this will shape his life as he gets older and becomes more aware of what is taking place. Now he just seems confused as to why his sister plays with such caution and awareness as he takes on every challenge as though he is indestructible.

Everyone is buckled into the car that Faith's father refuses to replace until Cal is old enough to know better than to spill everything he touches in it. Hopefully he will learn soon, or Cal might win before the car dies. The garage door opens to reveal another cold but sunny January day in Wisconsin. The warmth of the garage gives a false sense of how cold it really is outside, and Faith is wondering why she has to bundle in so many clothes, but the short walk from the curb to inside the school has her realizing that mother was right to wrap the scarf up just high enough so her eyes show through.

At the school door Faith's Aide, Mrs. Paul, is waiting to greet the trio and holds the door for them as to get out of the cold as quickly as possible.

Terri gives Faith a kiss and hug good-bye, and much to Cal's dismay, who would rather stay and play with all the kids; they leave to go grocery shopping.

It doesn't take Faith long to strip from the bundle of warm clothes and put them neatly in her space in the closet, and start gabbing with her friends in the classroom before her teacher, Mrs. Spenle, starts kindergarten class for the day.

~

It is shortly after lunch and Terri is cleaning up behind one of Cal's abstract food displays he has made with his lunchtime meal when she gets a call from Mrs. Spenle, and in a tone that Terri could recognize from being witness to many difficult situations with Faith, knew that she was hurt. The voice on the other end explained Faith had fallen and was injured quite severely and that she should come quickly. With much haste, Terri scooped up Cal and frantically made their way back to Greenfield Elementary two hours before the normal school day would end. Inside they found a brave little girl sitting in her chair doing her best to hold back the tears as her friends sat on the floor listening to a story Mrs. Spenle was reading. When Terri and Faith's eyes meet, Terri wants to cry but knows she can't. It will crush Faith and they would both break down and that would not help matters. Mrs. Paul explains how the fall happened, that Faith had stubbed her toe on the carpet getting up from her chair and lost her balance, and when she fell under her arm caught on the chair and she fell to her knee removing the skin from the knee and her under arm. The knee was bleeding and the skin was still rolled up under her arm and you could see the dermis layer below. Mrs. Paul had done such a good job of calming Faith down and protecting the wounds until Terri arrived. It was comforting to know Faith has put so much trust in Mrs. Paul.

Things had gone so well for half of the school year that many thought all the planning going into the school year was not necessary but in the

Living with Epidermolysis Bullosa

blink of an eye it all becomes necessary and the stark realization of how fragile Faith is, makes everyone who witnesses such an event pause and have a moment of self-realization of what is really important.

As Faith is leaving the classroom one of her friends gets up from the circle and goes over to Faith with a tear in her eye and gives Faith a hug and whispers in her ear I hope you feel better soon. Faith, with as much courage as she could muster, replies: I'll be fine, knowing full well the dressing changes on her newly acquired wounds will be painful for the next 10 to 14 days.

Terri carries Faith into the house now because the wound on the knee is starting to dry and making it hard for Faith to walk. Terri puts Faith on the couch and goes back for Cal. Terri knows she needs to occupy Cal before she can attend to Faith's needs and Faith also understands this and recognizes her mom's attempts to get Cal to sit in his high chair and eat chocolate pudding as nothing more than a momentary distraction, but Cal takes the bait and Terri now has about 5 minutes of uninterrupted time to attend to Faith.

By now Faith has got her pant leg up over the knee and has thoroughly inspected the wound. She is quick to let her mom know what she can't do and what is acceptable. With lots of tears and lots of persuading, mom has managed to cut the loose skin away from the wound and clean away the blood and apply a Mepilex bandage that is normally used on burn victims but works very well on EB patients also. Cal has completed his wall art of pudding and is ready to jump from his high chair so Terri will have to complete the aid to under the arm with a little boy pulling at her arm. This sore does not appear as bad as originally expected, but it proves to be a bothersome slow healer.

Faith soon settles in with some food her mom had made for her and starts watching her favorite shows on television Dora the Explorer or High School Musical or whatever is on Nickelodeon next. Getting to eat on the couch and watching her TV is little consolation for going through such an ordeal, but Faith makes it work. Faith knows her day has not yet run its course, that even though these wounds, as bad as they are, will still not eliminate the need to change the daily bandages on her feet to keep the sores from filling with bacteria and keeping the blisters on her feet under control.

When Faith's father gets home she gives him the full report on what happened and how it was an accident and that it was just something that could not be helped or foreseen. Through the entire explanation you can't help but notice Faith was more concerned about upsetting her friends and how helpful Mrs. Paul and Mrs. Spenle were and never once mention how bad it hurt or asking for an ounce of pity.

Once sometime ago, when Faith's bandage changes on her feet were not going so well, she asked her mom why she couldn't be normal, and her mom, with tears running down her face could only hug the little girl as strongly as she dare and say, you are normal. Faith couldn't bear to see her mom cry and never asked again. This is something I know Faith keeps inside her and recognizes situations where people are uncomfortable and she becomes a mediator to the situation. At her age it is a remarkable personality trait to show so strongly.

They all sit down to dinner with the evening news in the background. Faith manages to sit up to the table and eats with everyone, more so because she enjoys it most when the family is altogether at the table and she can have their full attention to tell her stories and what she has learned. After dinner Faith makes her best attempts to get out of her dressing changes and as much as her mother and father would like to say O.K., it just needs to be done to prevent infections. She agrees as long as her father holds her hand and Cal sits on his lap. Fortunately changes went well they took only about 20 minutes as opposed to 45 minutes if there are complications.

Faith's father makes a bowl of popcorn and they sit together to read a book as mom rocks Cal to sleep. Then it's off to bed and with a good night and an "I love you". That extraordinary little girl is back in her bed with the same grin she woke up with, thinking she is fooling everyone into her being a sleep with her eyes half open and giggling. Her parents, without saying anything, can tell they are both wishing tonight's dreams are happy ones. The extraordinary little girl soon falls asleep with the grin still on her face, as if she knows tomorrow is promised to her.

~

Living with Epidermolysis Bullosa

Just (find a way to) Do It!

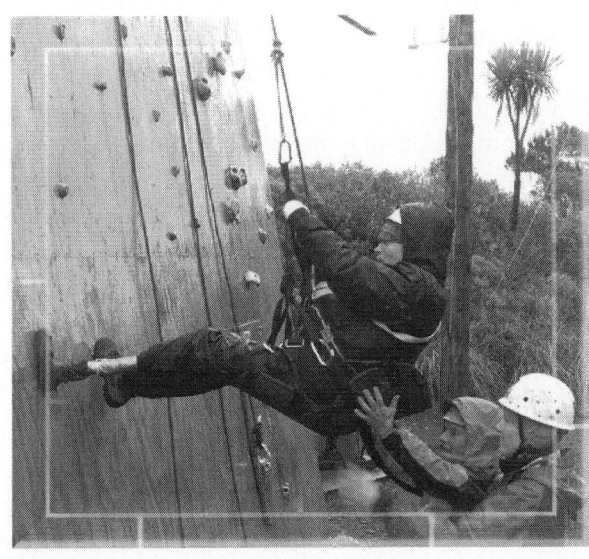

By Ashley W.
k.j.worthy@xtra.co.nz
Northland New Zealand

Ashley W is a young man who has RDEB. He lives in his own house on his parent's property in a small rural town in Northland New Zealand. As owner and DJ of the local community radio station, Ashley is well known and his sense of humor and zest for life means that things around him are never dull. Here Ashley shares some of his thoughts and adventures that keep him on the sunny side of EB life!

Hi my name is Ashley, I am 21 years old and I live in Northland New Zealand where I spend my days in a little old caravan running my own community radio station: Radio Waves 99.1FM. I have Recessive Dystrophic EB and unfortunately that means that the highs in my life need to be squeezed in around dressing changes, eye blisters, throat dilatations, hospital visits for surgeries and gastro feeds. But don't let this list of hardships depress you because my life is good!

I have been given the privilege of sharing with you some of my thoughts on EB. Read and enjoy but keep in mind that firstly and fore mostly I am a 21 year old male, and that I make every effort to ensure that EB takes a back seat!

From day one I have lived my life to the max. Just (find a way to) Do it has been the family motto. I'm the first to admit that living with EB has slowed me down considerably but hasn't stopped me.

When I'm not on air on my radio station I'm usually indulging my other passion, driving! I drive cars, tractors, boats, diggers, you name it, and I'll try and drive it. Driving is awesome, as it gets me out and about, and gives me independence. It is something that I can do well. Hey, I also love to party, have a few ales, cause moderate mayhem with my friends and basically do everything a normal, young, good-looking male does!

How do I do these things when EB has left me so disabled? Well, family and friends play a huge part in my life. I am always hanging out with my mates (mum's other sons, as she says) and it is with these very close friends that most of my adventures happen. Where there's a will there's a way and between us we find it. Adapt it, build it, change it, lift it, carry it, and push it. I'm the first to admit I would be lost without their help and because of this appreciation I try to work very hard on my friendships!

At first I was unsure what to write for this book, but luckily I'm a born optimist. I don't take time to dwell on the negative side of life in the EB lane so why write about it. Instead, I thought it would be fitting to share some of my most memorable adventures.

EB has given me many opportunities to meet great people and go to wonderful places but the highlights in my life have been closer to home.

My 15th birthday was the greatest day of my life!!! This was the day I got my driver's license. For my friends and I it was a day we had dreamed about, talked about and secretly practiced for, for several years! I had a serious decision to make two years earlier as I was unable to drive due to a deformed lower left leg. I was born with no skin on this leg and the constant breakdown and consequent scarring had left me without the power to push in the clutch and this was not on, not on at all! It took everyone a long time to come around to my idea. I knew that to get my driver's license my leg had to go!

I think at the time mum and dad were hoping I would give it two weeks and move on but I wanted to drive more than I wanted anything else in the world and after a year of meeting with doctors and specialists, researching amputations, and many big family debates, I won! I finally convinced everyone that amputation was the answer to all my problems and as my leg was painful and was of no use to me, I could only gain from having it removed.

Needless to say on the day of my 15th birthday I passed my driver's test with flying colors and have never looked back. Ha! Who says teenagers don't know their own mind! To this date, it has been the best decision I have ever made and I as well as being able to drive with my prosthesis, I can now even walk a bit too.

At this point I am going to introduce my good friends Nathan, Lyndon, Rory, and Shane. I am going to share with you a little story about our first encounter with cars and gravity: The day had been spent on Nathan's farm using the tractor to build a jump ramp for the hack around Austin 1300 car. Yes, his parents were away but we were acting responsibly. I did take precautions! I put on an extra jumper for padding (smart thinking aye?) I have to admit here that the thought of just watching did enter my mind fleetingly but no way was I missing out, so I joined the boys in the car for our first and last car jump.

If all went to plan, we would hone around the paddock to build up speed and then hit the ramp. On our calculations we would fly through the air in a movie style arch before making the perfect landing. We were off and going for gold. So far so good, then we hit the jump only to find that our calculations were somewhat off. It was us that went flying up; unfortunately, at the same time as the car came crashing down. Five heads came in sharp contact with the roof! Nothing broken. My mates had sore necks and heads for a week and I had all of the above plus a fair bit of skin to regrow! It just goes to show that you can't always believe what you see on the television!

My other love is boating. My baby is a 12ft tin dinghy with a 6hp outboard. We have adapted the throttle for me to use, as my hands are almost clubs now. I'm the Captain and as of right now give the orders, which are obeyed or not, depending on the crew's whim.

This day we had planned to explore the river ways around our town and had loaded the boat with all the essentials, coke, lollies, and chocolate, everything we needed to survive. We set off at a nice pace (full speed) to see where we would end up. After an hour of cruising we came across a tree that was partially submerged and blocking the river.

After much discussion we opted for the easy but somewhat stupid (appropriate for us) way round the problem, go over at full speed.

Yes you guessed it, I lost more skin. But hang on a minute; every EB adventurer knows that to go out without an emergency kit is foolish and foolishness is not one of my downfalls. A few major repairs and some paracetamol and things were back on track.

After the boys had spent the next hour trying to dig the boat free, we decided to call it quits and Nathan drew the short straw and walked the 2 hours home to get the van. He came driving through the farm to collect us and after much heaving, shoving and swearing, the boat, with Captain Ash still at the helm, was dragged up the side of a bank, loaded onto the van and driven home. A grand ending to a fun day!

In the last two years I've had the privilege of indulging my adventurous spirit even more. DEBRA NZ has run two amazing out-doors adventure camps and as well as meeting other teens with EB I have tried many new activities that have tested both my physical and mental skills. Using expertly adapted equipment to meet my EB needs, I've tried white water rafting, abseiling, rock climbing, gliding, and best of all skiing.

I love skiing! With thousands of extra bandages and a sit ski, I have learned to ski unaided and now can whiz (well, whiz in my books!) down the mountain on my own.

This is where mum gets weepy! Not because skiing is dangerous, she's hardened up to that after years of trying to dissuade me but, because she says she never dreamed her baby, born with such a serious skin condition, would ever be able to do something as exciting and adventurous as this.

What about your skin coming off I hear you ask? What about the dangers, the consequences, the recovery time? Is it really worth it?

Yes it is! Early on I learnt that with EB whatever you do has a price to pay, you have to weigh it all up. Sometimes it's a few small blisters, sometimes more. Once, I did a vast amount of damage, but no regrets, I made the choice.

Everyday there are a million EB reasons to stay in bed, feel sad, cheated, angry and ask why me? But I've decided that as no one knows what the future holds for me or for EB in general, I have no intention of just sitting around waiting to find out. I intend to live my life to the fullest!!

~

Living with Epidermolysis Bullosa

And We Go On

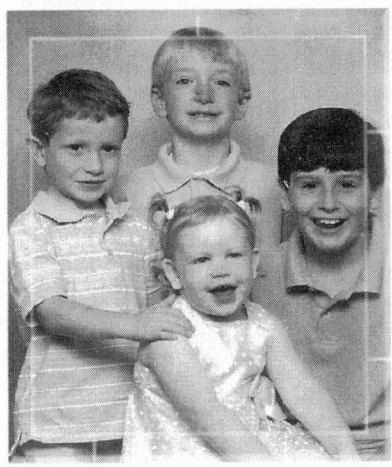

By Debby L.
lillydk@jmu.edu
Virginia, USA

Debby L. is the wife (Roy, Simplex), mother (Sarah, Simplex) and grandmother (Andrew Jordan, Recessive Dystrophic) of three EBers. They live in Virginia USA. This is her story of how EB is not an end but a beginning, a blessing not a curse. It is to show the life does go on and can be as full of hope and joy as you allow it to be.

When I met Roy in 1974, I was just coming out of a horrible and traumatic marriage. I was 20 years old and I had just done the one thing I promised myself I would never do, go back to my parent's house. I got a job at Westinghouse to try and make a life for my daughter, Paige and myself. That is where I met this funny little guy who changed my life. He was warm and caring and he made me laugh, something I thought I had forgotten how to do. Two years later, we got married.

When I first met him, I noticed that he walked slowly and sometimes had a slight limp but it just didn't seem important at the time. After a while, he finally told me that he got blisters on his feet and that it was because of a condition he inherited from his father. My dad gets blisters if he wears colored socks so again I thought "big deal". It wasn't until he actually showed me his feet that I understood how big a deal it was. However, by then, I was madly in love with the goofy little guy.

When we got married, we both wanted more children very much. We didn't think much about the blisters because it just didn't seem to happen very often and we just hoped for the best. After six miscarriages, we had Becky. While I was pregnant, wise guy said he hoped we had a little girl who looked like me and had his personality (he didn't think he would survive two people with my temper). What he got was a little girl who looked just like him and had MY personality. Ha! That will teach him to be careful what he wishes for!

Becky was perfect in every way. Sometimes, I would look at her and wonder how I had gotten so lucky. She was so strong, smart and healthy, so we put all thoughts of EB out of our minds. She sat up at 5 months and walked at 8. From the first step on, she ran and climbed wherever she went, good grief, nothing was safe.

I have always wanted a ton of kids so no one was surprised when I turned up pregnant at my six weeks checkup. Of course, the doctor read us the riot act but I didn't care; I was going to have another baby! I made it to 7 months and then in a flash it was all over. The problem is, my babies have very short umbilical cords, and the weight of the baby causes it to pull the cord loose, there is nothing that can be done once it starts. I didn't give up hope, I had Becky and I was sure there would be more.

My mother in law had a fit when she found out I was pregnant after Becky and one day she made me so mad that I said I would be pregnant again on Becky's first birthday if I wanted to! Remember what I said about being careful what you wish for? Well, I was pregnant on Becky's first birthday!

Sarah was born August 1. Roy was out on strike and money was tight but he had finally gotten his wish - a girl who looked like me and had his personality. Unfortunately, he had forgotten what a little brat he was as a child! Only one thing had us concerned when Sarah was born - she had a blister on her finger.

The doctor laughed it off saying he had seen it many times before and that she was destined to be a thumb-sucker. We checked her feet and they looked fine so again thoughts of EB were put away. Then when she was 4 days old I got her up one morning and noticed blood on her pajama feet. I took them off and the tops of her feet were covered with blisters.

It was only the beginning. Roy was devastated. He blamed himself and became determined to find a way to cure her. That's where the 12-year search for a doctor who could help started.

We went through thousands of dollars and so many doctors that I lost count. She became a guinea pig for every crack pot who thought he could make a name for himself. The "cures" ranged from massive doses of vitamin E that almost cost her life, to a plan to burn the skin off of her feet with a laser, the idea being that the new skin would grow in blister free. When she was 12, she said she had had enough and I supported her decision. Roy still believed that all we had to do was find the right doctor but I had finally faced the truth - there was no cure.

Sarah never let her feet stop her from what she wanted to do. We are a family of jocks and she was determined to be a part of it. I wanted so much to say no and not let her but she taught me that there was no point in keeping her alive if we weren't going to let her live. She played softball, basketball, ran track and cross-country. The price she paid was sometimes more than I could stand but I refused to let her see it. Whatever she wanted to try, I supported her even if it meant helping her change her shoes and socks at half time because the sound of the blood squishing in her shoes was upsetting the other players. I learned so much about the power of the human spirit from that little girl. Life went on.

The girls grew up and blisters were just a little part of our lives. Paige was the first to give us a grandchild and he was a beautiful little boy, Brian Lee. This was quite a thrill for me as I was one of three girls and had three girls myself. A BOY! Wow! Then Becky called to say she was pregnant. She and her husband were stationed at Fort Riley Kansas so I was concerned that we wouldn't get to see much of our new grandchild. When we went out to see them in November, she had an ultrasound done and he was very obviously a little boy. I feel in love right then and there and was determined to be there when he was born. When the call came that Becky was really in labor, I started calling the airport trying to get a flight. That's when I found out that there was a women's basketball tournament going on and it was impossible to fly into the entire state of Kansas! In steps my white knight, Roy, who volunteered to drive me straight through to Kansas -1105 miles one way (now can you see why I still love the old grump!).

We stopped about half way and were told there was something wrong with Andrew's skin. Roy and I both knew right then what it was but we had no idea the extent of the problem. We had always been told that it just involved the hands and feet. Well, we made it to Irwin Army hospital at 4AM on the 28th and there he was, swaddled and sleeping. I didn't have my glasses on so I couldn't see what everybody was making such a fuss about.

It wasn't until later that morning, during a bandage change, that I got my first lesson in what Epidermolysis Bullosa was really all about. It was overwhelming. He was missing all of the skin from his left foot, right hand and right thigh. There were blisters and scabs on his face and stomach. His little mouth was a disaster area.

That day became the first day of a long struggle to find a way to make a life for that precious little boy. He didn't want to suck and the doctor recommended that we not try to make him eat. When I asked if he meant for us to let him starve the doctor's answer - "If you love him you will" - was almost more than I could stand. But that man didn't know our family very well. It just made us more determined. We were told all about how malnutrition induced mental retardation and that was all it took. We went out and bought droppers and fed him by hand. He ate like a starving man, downing 6 ounces of formula in no time flat. That was when I made Andrew a promise that if he wouldn't give up, neither would I.

When Andrew was 5 days old we all went to Denver to see an EB Specialist. We had to strip him naked and they took pictures and told us what we already knew - this was for life and there was no cure. I watched my little girl that I had tried so hard to bring into this world face the facts of her son's life. She cried and then raised her head and I saw the look on her face. She wasn't going to give up either!

I guess it was easier for us having some experience with EB. Andrew's father and his parents just couldn't seem to get a handle on what this all meant. Like so many marriages that involved children with special needs, this one was doomed from the moment the doctor said the words "No cure". Mothers don't have the luxury of saying: "I can't deal with this."

The following October we then became a household where EBers actually outnumbered non-EBers. Life became a daily battle to deal with whatever new thing EB threw at us. But it was so worth it to watch that delightful little boy grow and thrive.

At work I had access to a computer so I decided to try to find some help on the Internet. I found the DebRA website and while it had some interesting facts, it didn't seem to help much in the day-to-day life of raising an EB child. I checked back every now and then but didn't seem to find much. Then one day in April, I found a website owned by a woman named Silvia who had a little boy named Nicky who had EB.

When I saw the first picture of that beautiful little boy, I touched the screen and called him my little Pooh Bear. I was hooked! Madly in love with a little boy I thought I would never get to know. I signed the guest book and thought well that's that, but at least I can go and visit the website everyday and be reassured that there are others out there. I was surprised and confused when I got an email from this Silvia about walking with sorrow. Boy, I wrote her back in a heartbeat letting her know there was no sorrow connected with Andrew, I would not allow it! She wrote back letting me know that she had sent the poem looking for my reaction. She invited me to join a group of 8 other women who were raising EB children. That was the day everything changed. We were not alone anymore! I don't know if Silvia will ever realize how much she means to my family and me. I just know that I thank God for her every day. I have met so many wonderful people that have become such a precious part of my life.

Finally, Becky decided that it was time to go out on her own. She and Andrew moved about 20 minutes away. Some days I miss him so much it hurts but I know it is best for them to have their own lives. Brian (the oldest grandson) went to live with her. She has remarried and has a beautiful little girl, Rylyn Maeve. Her husband has his own little boy, Michael, so now I am Nanny to four.

Sarah is a Math teacher and about to be married so it is just Roy and I here. We have both the boys (and sometimes Rylyn Maeve and Michael) on the weekends so there is still never a dull moment.

At first, I just couldn't understand. Why me? Then Andrew began to question why God had done this to him. I tried to explain that God wanted him to be special but I could tell that answer was wearing kind of thin. Then last fall we had an amazing experience. At the Buddy Ball (baseball that accommodates a player's different needs) banquet a mother came up and told us how grateful she was for Andrew. That day her autistic son had asked if he was going to see his friend Andrew. It was the first time in his life he had acknowledged another person as his friend. When we told Andrew he looked at me and said, "Well, Nanny, it was all worth it." That is when I realized that I was right all along. God had made him special; EB was a blessing, not a curse, and Andrew was perfect. For anyone to go through as much as he does and then believe it to be worth it because it helped another human being is special beyond all imagining and that I am blessed enough to even know such a person is the very meaning of true joy.

Well, that is the story of my life so far. It has been a wild ride and I can't wait to see what is next. Yes there were non-EB related events in my life but somehow they just don't seem to be as important as I thought they were at the time. EB is a force to be dealt with every minute of every day. There is never a moment when the person with EB or the people who love them can just "forget" and act like life is "normal". But we go on because that is what we must do. We make jokes and laugh and learn from one another and we go on. We cry and pray and pray some more and we go on. We believe and we go on. And we go on.

~

Living with Epidermolysis Bullosa

Living with an Angel

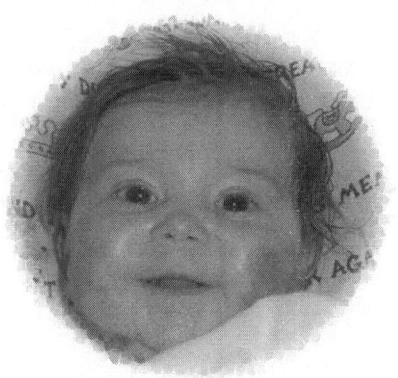

By Jennifer L.
skihome1@aol.com
Wisconsin, USA

Jennifer L. is the mother of Sophia, who lost her battle in 2002 to Junctional Herlitz EB. After 18 months of DNA testing, Sophia's mutations were identified, which allowed testing on her older sister Amelia and baby sister Olivia. Both of her sisters are EB free and not carriers of this dreaded disease. Her story shares the 9 months of love, devotion, lessons learned, and heartache in fighting for Sophia's life...

On Monday night May 7, 2001 at 9:52 PM, one of the most beautiful children in the world entered this earth weighing in at 7 pounds 13 ounces. After a seemingly normal pregnancy and much anticipation, Sophia Maria blessed us with her presence and officially became a member of our little family.

When the Doctor held her up and pronounced that we had a little girl my heart overflowed with joy and love for this beautiful baby. Our 2 1/2 year old daughter Amelia was certain the whole pregnancy that she was having a baby sister and her dream came true.

Sophia was so gorgeous and took our hearts the moment we saw her. However, immediately after birth, the doctor and nurses immediately noticed that something was not "right" with her. She had open blisters on all of her fingernails, a few on her toenails, and open wounds on the back of her wrists. She had her umbilical cord wrapped around her neck, which luckily caused her no damage, and waited a little while before taking her first breath with a little assistance from oxygen.

While the nurses were washing her up I looked across the room and saw her open fingertips and asked what was wrong and no one had an answer but said they would have a specialist come up later and have a look at her.

That night Sophia and I slept together in bed snuggling as tight as we could and who would have known that from that moment on our lives had changed forever as we knew it.

The following morning her pediatrician came to the hospital for her first checkup and after looking her over commented that he thought she may have Epidermolysis Bullosa (EB), but would need to send us to a specialist to confirm. I had no idea what this term meant and how it would turn our world upside down with the battle we would face for our beautiful daughter's life.

So, instead of a typical happy homecoming, 36 hours after Sophia's birth we were discharged and sent over to Children's Hospital of Milwaukee to meet with a team of dermatologists.   Soon it was confirmed that yes, indeed, she had this dreaded disease, but the severity of it would be unknown until a skin biopsy was complete. They took her biopsy, provided us with some EB literature, and informed us that in a worst case scenario the disease would attack her respiratory system and take her life.

From that instant I felt like a deer in headlights and could not believe what I was hearing. I grabbed her and hugged her as tight as I could and stated that a disease I had never heard of was not going to take my child and we would fight this disease with every ounce of our strength and energy. How could this happen to my daughter? I had Amelia and she was perfectly healthy and my husband and I knew of no one in the family history that had ever had this genetic disease, let alone heard of it.

Sophia's first month was pretty wonderful. She had gained almost 2 pounds and had only a few new blisters here and there, but nothing too severe. She was a very alert and attentive little girl and was already tracking things at just a few days old. She loved to be held, kissed, and cuddled; she was a very calm baby and so sweet. She loved to be around her big sister and would instantly stop crying the second she heard Amelia's voice and turn to whatever direction she heard her.

On the 12th of June I had to take her to the pediatrician because she had a cold for a few days and was just not feeling "right." She was a little congested and was having a hard time eating and breathing at the same time, and would end up spitting and coughing a few seconds after she ate.

She had lost 1/2 pound, which I was not surprised to hear, but everything else seemed okay. Her lungs sounded clear and she had been running no fever. So I had her sleep sitting up in her car seat or elevated in her crib, the same thing that I had done for her older sister as an infant, but not knowing all the while that this was the beginning of the relentless battle against this evil disease.

Two weeks later we went back to the doctor because she was still not gaining weight, she was congested and coughed after her feeds. We tried changing her nipples on the bottles, increased her caloric intake and monitored her weight for the next three weeks.

On July 22, 2001 we had Sophia christened and she looked like a sweet and precious Angel in her christening gown. She was so beautiful and we were all so in love with her. I knew then that something dreadful was coming and not really sure what it was.

Eight days later we had to take Sophia to the emergency room because she was so lethargic and not eating anything and had this horrible cough that just did not sound "right." The staff ran some chest x-rays on her and noticed that her right upper lobe on her lung was collapsed and said that it was possible pneumonia. Sophia was instantly admitted and IV antibiotics were started. My husband and I were almost relieved to hear that it could be something "fixable" and thought everything would be better in a few days.

The next morning the infectious disease specialist came in and explained to us that he felt it was not pneumonia, but rather aspiration and that she may need a feeding tube (g-tube) placed to help her. The next week in the hospital was so tiring and emotional and every question led to another test, which led to more decisions for Sophia. By the end of the week it was decided, after a barium swallow study, that she had severe aspiration and was burning her calories faster than she could swallow them. After discussing it at length with her specialists, we decided to have her g-tube placed three days later.

We scheduled a care conference with all of her specialists and reviewed at length how Sophia's tube was to be placed in the least evasive way to prevent further skin and internal damage based on her fragility and current condition.

We stressed how Sophia was a very precious child and that there was no room for error with her. When the staff wheeled her away for surgery I was a mess; for the first and only time, Sophia was out of my control and this drove me crazy. We were Sophia's number one advocates and for the next few hours we had to trust the doctors and pray that all would go smoothly for her.

Sophia came through surgery okay, a few extra blisters here and there, but overall all went well. They wheeled her in her room and I ran next to her bed and she opened her eyes for a second, looked at me and smiled as if to tell me that things were going to be okay. Oh, how I loved to look into those gorgeous eyes of hers. Her eyes were the window to so much and spoke volumes.
Everyone who met her always commented on how beautiful her eyes were.

After a few days of observation we went home and tried to have as "normal" of a life as we could again. Sophia started to gain weight slowly and was trying her hardest to regain the strength that she once had. She had her first three teeth cut through on the 19th of September and was a champ! She smiled that morning as if she was trying to show them off and was starting again to grab her toys and have a little extra energy.

We were very optimistic even though it had been confirmed that she was diagnosed with Junctional EB after a second biopsy and just loved her with every breath that we had. She had even started to coo and would carry on numerous "conversations" with anyone that would listen. She was a very content and happy baby despite all that she was dealing with. Sophia endured quite a bit of damage during her hospital stay and as hard as we tried to heal her, the more her skin just seems to break down.

Late in the evening on September 22, I heard Sophia "breathing" in a very loud and unusual fashion and ran to her bedside to find her struggling for air. This terrified me to the bone and I awoke my husband to call 911 and explain to them Sophia's disease and the problems she was enduring. Within minutes, two ambulances, two police units and plenty of lights in the middle of the night arrived at our home. Before the medical technicians could even touch her I had to explain as quickly as I could what EB was and what could/could not be done to Sophia. I was so scared and shaking as I held her and tried to help calm her through her tough bouts.

Through it all Sophia always continued to amaze me. She remained so calm and just looked at me as if to tell me she was trying to work through it and not worry me. She will always be one of the most amazing people I will ever meet and am so proud to be known as her Mother. We went on to the emergency room and this time it was thought that she had croup due to her breathing condition and her positive response to steroid treatments. We were sent home after explaining very firmly that the hospital was the worst place for Sophia due to potential infection and comfort issues; the staff agreed and discharged us eight hours after admission.

The next month went okay. Sophia's breathing was a constant up and down and on the 21st of October we were once again admitted to PICU for a few days with no official diagnosis except for a guess that this hideous disease had entered our daughter's airway. Two days after being discharged from the hospital we were back again in the middle of the night and Sophia was fighting her hardest to just relax and work through whatever was annoying her airway. Her ENT doctor confirmed by x-rays that her airway had narrowed and we needed to discuss the option of a tachometry.

I was once again heartbroken that no matter what we did and how hard we fought this hideous disease it did not care and was laughing at us as we tried our hardest to save our sweet little Sophia.
The next few days were a constant extreme between down and further down. My husband and I, along with her specialists, discussed at length what would be the best decision for Sophia. I wanted to help her in every way that we could, but after praying and discussing we opted that a tachometry was not the best thing for Sophia. We all knew that Sophia was very weak and fragile to begin with, and just had a really bad feeling that she would not make it through the surgery.

There were many rough nights and many hours of crying over why this was attacking such a sweet little Angel and all we could do was love her and make her as comfortable as possible. Infections continuously attacked her both internally and externally. If we thought we had cleared an infection up it was only for a short time and would reappear a few days later stronger and more immune to our current antibiotic schedules. We tried numerous antibiotics and were admitted a few times to the hospital to help clear things up, but as soon as one aspect of this disease was being treated there were four-five evils waiting in the wings laughing at us.

Sophia was so strong through everything and fought as hard as she did because she knew she was so loved and so much a part of our lives. Amelia told me that she had an idea on how to help Sophia - we should put Sophia back in my tummy where she was safe. Oh how I would have jumped at such an option. Amelia was so amazing with her and loved her with a passion that is indescribable. She was her protector and the sister's shared a bond that I will never be able to express in words.

Sophia loved to hear her sister and Amelia loved to help her sister.

December was another tough month and all we could do was keep ourselves focused on Sophia's comfort. Her doctors, nurses, and specialists were so wonderful and loving with her and our family. They always listened to what we wanted and helped us work through tough issues. We tried numerous blood transfusions to help bring up Sophia's iron levels, but as soon as we brought it up it started its slide down. We developed numerous pain medication schedules to keep her comfortable and it seemed that every week her pain elevated and we increased her morphine and methadone intake to keep her comfortable.

EB is evil and not only did it attack our daughter's skin and her internal organs, but it also attempted to strip her of her beauty and cheerful personality. EB robbed her of so much and the only thing that we could "control" was her pain discomfort. She used to have the brightest look in her eyes and all you could see now was discomfort and sadness. Sophia could no longer smile and was sleeping more hours in a day than awake and it wasn't from her medications, but from the exhaustion of fighting and trying to live with EB.

We made it through the holidays and I was so thankful that Sophia was there to share them with us. She tried her hardest to be happy and would never complain. Diaper changers were now a 45-minute procedure, bath time was 2 1/2 hours long, and just picking her up to love her was a very slow action. Her skin was over 85% broken down and shedding off whenever healing tried to start. You never saw her get mad or cry over all of this though; she would just look at me with intense concentration in those big beautiful eyes and try her hardest not to cry. She was being brave for me - what an amazing little girl.

The last week in January I knew that Sophia's condition was somehow turning worse. She now had various infections and was on antibiotics for three weeks and things were moving nowhere in the positive. She was sleeping more and just not herself. On the 29th of January we had our Priest perform confirmation rights with Sophia and say a few prayers with us; I could not believe it had come to this. We fought so hard for her and did all that we could for her, but EB did not care, it just continued to torture my beautiful little girl.

The morning of February 9, 2002, was like any other morning. Sophia stayed up a little longer in the morning before her nap and was taking in so much of Amelia talking to her. I laid her down for a nap around noon and kissed her and hugged her and told my Angel that I loved her and was so proud of her. I set her feeding machine up while she fell asleep and left her home with my husband so that Amelia and I could go out for a few hours for the first time in months.

Her feeding was complete about an hour later and Ernie ran in her room to turn off the beeping alarm so it would not wake her up. As he was shutting the machine off she awoke for a second and looked at him like she always did when she heard someone in the room and immediately went back to sleep. A few minutes later I returned home and ran upstairs to check on Sophia and as I entered her doorway I knew at that moment she was gone. She looked so gorgeous and was the most relaxed I had ever seen her. I ran to her and picked her up and hugged her so tight and kissed her all over, she hurt no more and no one could hurt her ever again.

Her pediatrician and home nurse, as promised months before, immediately came over to confirm her passing. We all held her and hugged her and thanked God for easing her pain and struggle and taking her while she slept. We made clay prints of her hands and feet and kept her at home with us for a few hours to just love her and say our good-byes to her. Amelia held her and said to me "Look Mama she's not crying anymore when I hold her."

Sophia was and always will be the bravest person I have ever known. She was and always will be my second born and baby girl. She had the most incredible eyes and sweetest smile. Anyone that got to meet her or know her was lucky. EB is rare, but a child as sweet and beautiful as Sophia is even rarer. She was loved intensely and taught us and so many others so much about life. The world is a much better place after Sophia's presence. We will forever love and miss her and know that she knew we will forever be proud of her and her fight was so intense because she was loved so much.

As I sit here five years later and reflect on all that has happened in the past few years I am so thankful for Sophia and all that she shared with us. There isn't a day that goes by that we don't talk about her or think of her. She will always be a part of our family and a dearly loved and missed sister.

Although Sophia went through so much I know that her life with us was happy because we loved her so much and did everything for her and not our own selfish reasons. She is a continuous inspiration to us and so many other people. Sophia taught us that life is a gift and one that we should treasure no matter how long or short it may be.

I take solace in knowing that one day we will be joined together in heaven and look forward to that joyful reunion.

~

Tears for Dillin

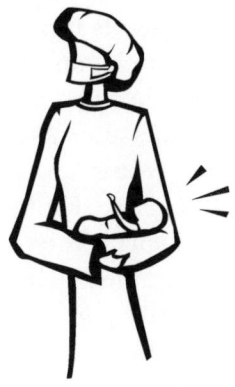

By Connie P.
copwife12@cox.net
Louisiana, USA

Connie is the mother of an RN Nurse in labor and delivery at a local hospital and met baby Dillin (with EB) while volunteering to rock babies in the NICU unit.

I would like to relate my first and only personal experience of a child with EB. I am the mother of two healthy grown girls, with my youngest being a Registered Nurse in labor and delivery at a local hospital. It was during her school semester working at the hospital that she discovered the need for volunteers to rock babies in the NICU unit. It was something I had never done before and eagerly put in my application and went through the necessary steps to begin rocking babies.

On one of the rather slow days that I was in the NICU, there was a nurse that I had become quite familiar with, and she asked if I had ever been in the back room yet. I said that I had not but I was willing to visit and give it a try. She explained that the little boy in the back room was quite a sad story.

And so began my relationship with Dillin.

Dillin was about two months old when I first met him. The very first time I saw him he had blisters all over his little body and was greased down and wrapped in bandages. I was instructed that I could not touch his skin; that I had to wear a long sleeve paper gown and rubber gloves anytime I picked him up. Dillin apparently inherited EB from his mother, who was 17 years old at the time of his birth. She walked in one time, looked at him, and walked away.

She has never been back or even inquired about Dillin.

Dillin's EB was so severe that it apparently affected his brain, hearing and sight. Many tests were run upon his small body. He has a feeding tube in his stomach so they can feed him. It was determined that he has brain damage. It was also determined that he has hearing loss, but we don't know whether it is a total hearing loss. He also has some sight problems and we believe that he possibly sees shadows but not much more. The nurse explained to me that she has been a nurse for 29 years and this is the first time she has seen this disease. It was surprising to me how many nurses had never even heard of EB. That made me realize the rarity and also that there must be a reason I was introduced to this little baby.

None of this stops me from visiting and holding him each time I go to the hospital. The first time I saw him, I walked away so upset, but looking for answers. That is when I discovered the EB website and signed up for regular updates. There was even a poem on the website that I printed and put on Dillin's crib.

Dillin is now 9 months old and still in the NICU unit. He has become a ward of the state and has had several prospective foster parents visit him, but no one will take him home. He was to be placed in a state home for care, but they have been unable to locate a facility that will take him.
It just breaks my heart!

He has grown so much and, in my mind at least, he does see and hear and, of course, feels the pain! Unfortunately, as he gets older and with the problems that he has, the potential of someone adopting him grows slimmer.

I wanted my R.N. daughter, who works in labor and delivery at the same hospital, to meet Dillin and brought her to NICU one day to do so. He was lying on his back, half asleep, and I said his name. He then opened his eyes and turned in our direction. My daughter said: "Mom, he knows your voice". When I hold him now, he even sometimes laughs. When I turn on the mobile on the bed above his head, he turns his head to look. This is why we believe he does see something!

The first time I saw him smile was the first time I held him at about two months old. All greasy and wrapped in bandages with sores and blisters, he was sleeping and smiled! I absolutely fell in love with him, so innocent and unaware of his dilemma. Unfortunately, I am not in a position to be able to take Dillin home. If I was financially secure and did not have to work, I would bring him to my home in a heartbeat and hire a nurse to help care for him.

I know he will not have much of a life, but I want to make a difference in his life as much as I can. Being that he is prone to infections, if and when he ever leaves the hospital, a state facility and state workers will not tend to him in the same careful manner that the nurses in NICU are doing. As one nurse explained to me, he would probably get an infection from improper care and eventually die. This absolutely broke my heart! This poor baby didn't ask to even be born and yet he has this disease to deal with and no one to love and care for him!

I want people to know about EB. I signed the Wound Care Bill petition online and also had all my family and friends do the same. I have spoken to anyone who will listen and I tell them about Dillin and this horrible disease.

All my friends and family continue to ask for updates on Dillin's condition. When I go to the NICU unit, the nurses always ask me if I'm going to visit my little guy.

I don't know what Dillin's future holds but I intend to be part of his life, holding, rocking, singing and talking to him for as long as I can.

I know that one day he will no longer be part of my life, but I have learned so much from this experience and he will always be in my heart.

I have searched for answers and, of course, the reasons are bigger than we are and we will never understand them. I have shed tears for Dillin but it warms my heart to hold him and see him smile and be comforted. I will continue my efforts to educate people about EB and keep updated on this horrible disease. I will also keep in my prayers all the children born with this disease and hope they have someone to love and care for them.

~

EB is Not Easy - But You Can Learn to THRIVE!

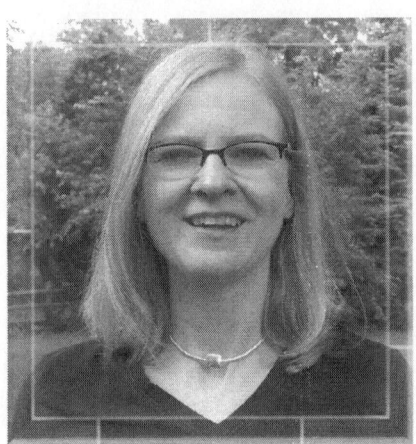

By Gretchen M.
morsegre@msu.edu
Michigan, USA

Gretchen M. is a 39 year-old woman with EB Simplex with Junctional variants. Between her EB and a family tragedy (and a difficult link between the two), she has used her pain to re-build her life into something that can better help her, and many others.

I was born on a Monday, August 14, 1967. My mother tells me that the birthing process tore almost 1/2 of the skin off of my body. Doctors were baffled, as they had not seen this before. It wasn't until weeks later, when an intern was making rounds and saw me that he was able to share with other doctors his experience seeing an EB baby at another hospital, and thus, a preliminary diagnosis was made.

I spent my first month of life in the hospital in an incubator, with very little human touch, as I was so fragile. Mom visited the hospital when she could, but she also had my brother who was two at the time. He was EB-free, as is the rest of the family. The only possible record of EB in the family is in a family bible on my father's side, which makes reference to an infant dying of "Eczema" several generations back. It is possible that baby had EB and they just didn't know what to label it.

My mom was not happy with my care and treatment and seeming lack of information the nurses at the hospital had, and made the decision to take me home and care for me herself. She did this around the clock, with no relief until a friend finally came and asked to be trained in how to take care of me, so my mother could get some rest.

I spent the first year buck-naked, as clothes would stick to the open skin or create new blisters and erosions. I was laid in on a stack of diapers, and the house was turned up to 80 degrees in order to keep me warm, without contact. When I had to go to the doctor, I was placed in a cardboard box lined with cotton, on the front seat of the car.

After my first year, clothes began to be somewhat more possible. In spite of all the troubles with my skin, I was labeled a "happy baby". Because of my EB, my parents decided to adopt their third child, and became the proud parents of Rochester, New York's first bi-racial adoption.

As I grew into toddler-doom, my parents held their breath when I took my first steps, roughhoused with my brothers, and sometimes fell. By school age, it was apparent that riding the bus and going to school were potential "dangers" in my frail condition. I was fortunate that my Dad was an elementary Art Teacher, and I could ride back and forth to school with him, and attend regular classes under his watchful eye. I cherish our rides together and him turning me loose in his glorious art room before and after school every day.

I never did take a gym class. Other kids thought I was "lucky", but I wanted more than anything to participate, and be "normal". Instead, I went to the library and "helped" the librarian with various projects. I was really well coordinated and would have loved to have tried my hand at gymnastics, softball or basketball.

There were many times kids made fun of me, calling me "bubbles", and other various insults. The staring almost felt worse; I often felt myself crawl deep inside, hiding from the embarrassment of those eyes penetrating my wounds.

There were a few days that the pain was too unbearable to go to school in the first place, or, I couldn't walk because of the blisters on my feet. There were other days that I had to be excused to the nurse's, and make the phone call to have my mom pick me up because the pain was intolerable.

My first two years of school were eased by the fact that I had two wonderful teachers. Mrs. Feller was my Kindergarten teacher, and greeted me the first day with special scissors she had found, that would be easier on my hands. She sometimes held me on her lap, and I could tell she truly cared for me. I still visit Mrs. Feller today!

I remember vividly an experience in first grade, with my wonderful teacher Mrs. Maciaszek. She was so caring and protective. We had a fire drill one day, and as she was instructing all the other students to form a line to walk outside, she gathered me up and placed me on her hip. We processed outside. I had bad blood blisters on my thigh that day, and the jostling of her walking painfully tore them open. Even worse than the physical pain, was seeing the gooey red smear on her beautiful cream suit after she put me down. I will never forget that.

As I got older, adapting to issues of pain, clothing, shoes and all the other things that came with EB became more routine, but never easy. One place I found comfort was in music. From the third grade on, I picked up every instrument I could get my hands on, and loved learning them.

I tried to appear as "normal" as possible and tried things like downhill skiing, roller-skating and hiking. There would be horrible blisters for 2-4 weeks afterwards, but it somehow felt "worth it" as I was able to experience those activities.

As I matured and went through puberty, the EB symptoms improved somewhat. I also began having many different little surgeries for the removal of dysplastic nevi. I still have those removals to this day.

High school was a furthering of my musical activities, and I knew that music would be my major in college. I was pleased to be allowed to attend college away from home, and the school was small enough, that I could navigate to and from classes most of the time.

I pursued music through three degrees, ultimately ending up with a Doctorate. I had a frenzied schedule of teaching at small colleges and playing in Symphonies throughout Michigan. However, the schedule and the demand of playing were taking its toll. I never seemed to have much muscle strength or endurance, and performances were always riddled with fear about having the strength to get through them. Often, there would be great amounts of pain in addition to the strength issues. The tissues in the back of my throat would tear and/or develop ulcers. My lips seemed to pull away from my gums after a lot of playing, causing searing pain. And then there were the fingertip blisters from the keys of the instrument. I pushed and pushed and pushed, as music was all I knew, and where I had established my identity. The thought of doing something else was unbearable.

In 1997, I received the shocking news that my younger adopted brother had gotten strung out on cocaine and had attacked my parents while they slept. He killed my father, and left my mother for dead. It turned life upside down.

The last ten years have been very difficult, and also has been a time of intense exploration and growth. In pursuing counseling for the family tragedy, I finally have dealt with some of the more personal issues of the EB and how it has impacted my life. For starters, I felt that if I had not had EB, my parents would probably have had another biological child, and we wouldn't have had the problems with my adopted brother, and my father would be here today. It was hard for a while to not be really angry at my health and the EB. I was also angry that my body was unable to keep up with the demands of a full-time music career, and was devastated at the thought of letting go of that dream. I was also angry about the energy that I spend in every single movement of the day, to ensure that I perform every motion with the utmost care, to not damage my skin or tissue. How I hold a fork, how I open a door, how I pick up and carry things, what clothes and shoes I wear (and how many articles of clothing and shoes are un-wearable - who the heck invented bras, anyway?), how far I walk, how I place my foot for each and every step the list is endless. And then, no matter how hard I try, there are always unforeseen injuries every day, from bumping the skin unexpectedly, to slipping concentration and not gripping something properly, causing tearing or blistering...

Then there are those days that for whatever reasons my skin feel full and painful, and I know that walking, long periods of sitting, clothing contacts, and anything I do with my hands will be a big challenge. Sometimes, by the end of the day, my hands are so sore I can't even get undressed without great physical pain, and certainly a lot of extra time and effort (and swearing!).

The impact of not having been touched much as a newborn has surely been a struggle in my conflicted feelings about touch, closeness and intimacy. Though I have made great strides with this, there is always a part of me that will be on guard, I think.

I could tell many stories about my experiences with doctors, from Dermatologists to surgeons to general practitioners, regarding their lack of awareness about EB, and their insensitivities to dealing with the medical and psychological implications of it. There were many times that medical situations were even greatly jeopardized by their ignorance. It surely makes those who go the extra mile to research and understand both my skin and me stand out.

So, there has been hardship, there has been anger, and there has been bitterness. However, EB has given me gifts as well. Living with fragile skin has helped me to understand some of the difficulties that others face, as well. Though it was painfully difficult to let go of my dreams of playing music full time, it ultimately occurred to me that music is a choice people choose whether or not to listen to, learn, or play music. There are many other things in life people do not choose, like illness, tragedy, abuse, learning disabilities, race, and a multitude of other difficulties.

I wanted to be able to help others to deal with the things in life that they hadn't chosen, and were stuck with. There were doctors, physical therapists and people in the mental health profession that had made a huge difference in my being able to cope with what I was dealing with. I wanted to be able to provide that compassion and understanding for others who were faced with difficult things.

I was fortunate enough to have Psychiatrist and Social Worker friends with their own clinic. They knew my situation, and also my interest in the brain, learning styles, and computers. They had learned about a new treatment for emotional and learning disorders called Neurofeedback. They paid for my training and offered me a job at their clinic.

I now use EEG equipment to help diagnose and improve people's cognitive and emotional difficulties. This job has been very rewarding, as I truly enjoy my work with each client and whatever they bring in to the office. I enjoy the challenge of trying to understand the various hardships each of them face, and trying to help them through on various levels. I am truly grateful to my friends for giving me the opportunity to help others and to help my body and spirit by being in an environment that is much more soothing to me physically and emotionally. I still play professionally and also teach, and will continue to do so as long as I am able, physically.

If given the chance to have my EB cured, I would surely take it. But I can now appreciate what it has taught me about life. I now look at the limitations I have more realistically and try not to ignore them and take on things that will cause me further injury. I am also grateful for the things I CAN do! But mostly, having EB has taught me that it is possible to thrive, no matter what you are dealt. I am forever grateful for those that took the time and patience to help me, and am happy to be in a field where I can provide the same understanding for others facing difficult illness and circumstances.

~

My Life Was Heartache!

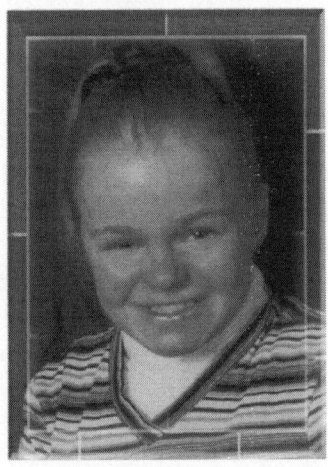

By Jennifer D.
Florida, USA

Jennifer was born on December 14th, 1979 in Wilmington, Delaware with the Recessive Dystrophic form of EB called Hallopeau-Siemens. She lived with her mom until August 1997, and then went to live with her grandma Shirley and her father Richard. She passed away on May 18th, 2005 due to kidney problems. She is survived by her beloved grandmother and caregiver, Shirley, her father, Richard, her sister Jodi and her brother, Anthony.

Once upon a time, there was this baby girl that was born in 1979 in Wilmington, Delaware, she had all of her fingers and all of her toes, but there was something not right with her skin. She had no skin on her left leg and also no skin on her stomach, and she had some blisters.

Nobody knew what this was until they had the Doctors come from A.I. Dupont Institute for Children in Wilmington Delaware. It took the Doctors three days to diagnose her with Epidermolysis Bullosa. I bet you would love to know her name: the little precious baby is Jennifer.

The words Epidermolysis Bullosa did not seem like they belonged to the English language when they told her Mother Joanne, her father Richard and her Grandmother. After they diagnosed Jennifer with EB, she was in the hospital for three or four months in isolation to guard against infection. They needed to teach Jennifer's mother how to take care of the wounds that she had and the blisters that would appear after a slight bump or scrap of the skin. The skin was very fragile. The nurses were really good about teaching Jennifer's mother how to change the bandages and keep the wounds nice and clean.

A year had passed and Jennifer was going to have a little sister. She was born in the same town and the same hospital that Jennifer was born in. The Doctors where afraid that Jodi would have EB as well, but she did not, that was good news for the family. One year later the girl's mother Joanne, was pregnant with her son Anthony by a different father, so she had three kids to take care of.

Nothing much was said about Anthony's father. Joanne was a very busy mother, not only did she have three babies, but also one had a very rare skin disorder and she had to teach herself a lot about Epidermolysis Bullosa. She had to constantly watch Jennifer and change her bandages every day. Joanne had to grind Jennifer's food because she could barely swallow. This was in the early eighties, before DebRA was founded, so there was no one to help Joanne.

After Jennifer and Jodi where born, their father Richard tried to help their mother, but she did not want their father anywhere near the girls. He wanted to help her because he loved his two baby girls, but Joanne kept their daddy away from them, so Jennifer and Jodi grew up without knowing their own father, they thought that their mother's boyfriends were their fathers (she had more than one). Joanne did not correct their thinking and let the girls believe that.

As the years went on, Joanne was getting abusive, mentally, physically and emotionally with Jodi, and then she started to be abusive with Jennifer.

Anthony was mommy's little boy and was rarely abused in any way. Jodi and Jennifer's Grandmother Shirley wanted to get custody of the girls because she knew Joanne was abusing them. She was so afraid for them that one day she called

Child Protective Services, but they did not do a thing to the mother; they kept the girls there, and went back to tell Shirley that they couldn't do anything because there was no sign of abuse. What is strange is that they also told Shirley to call them if she did not think that they would be okay in the home with their mother. It made no sense. Things went from bad to worse at this point. Joanne found out who called Child Protective Services on her, and from then on she didn't want the girls'

Grandmother to find out where they lived. When their Grandmother found them, Joanne would move. This went on for a few years.

At this point Jennifer was 8 years old, Jodi was 7 and their brother was 6. The girls knew that Anthony was their half brother, but they never told anyone, they loved him very much. Jennifer, being born with EB, had to grow up fast because of it, and was smarter than a normal 8 year old would be. Jodi and Jennifer were very close and they always would be.

One night Jodi told Jennifer that Gary (one of their mother's boyfriends) was sexually abusing her; this went on for years before she told her. Jennifer told her sister that they had to tell their mother that this was happening, but this was hard because their mother was physically abusing her already. In the end, Jennifer and Jodi told their mother, but she did not believe them at first. She got very angry with Jodi because she was doing that "to her". Jodi did not know that this was wrong; she was a little innocent girl at that time. Joanne was even getting worse with the physically abuse with Jodi. Nobody knew why she was like this just with Jodi and some with Jennifer. Jodi also told her teacher and the teacher called Child Protective Services who then investigated. A few weeks later Joanne called the Police and told them what was happening and they told her to bring Jodi to the Police station so they could talk with her about what Gary did to her. The hospital also examined her. Finally they charged him with sexual abuse, so he went to jail and served 8 years of the 20 that he was sentenced. He got out early because of good behavior. It's still unthinkable that they would release a sexual abuser!!

After that, Joanne must have said to herself: "Well, Gary will not be getting out of jail, so I have to go find me another man that will abuse my kids!" She may have not said this out loud, but her actions sure showed it.

Joanne was single for a while, and then comes along this guy, Robbie; he was no better than the other guy that was in jail. Joanne and Robbie only knew each other for a week and they wanted to get married, so they did behind everyone's back. Joanne did not even tell her own kids!!

Jodi, Anthony and Jennifer were living in Anthony, Florida; they had a nice 4-bedroom 2-bath trailer. Robbie did move in after they got married. Jodi's room and Jennifer's room were right across from each other, and Jenn would keep her door open because she had a very bad feeling about this guy that her mother was with.

Jenn was 14 years old, Jodi 13, and Anthony was 12 at this time. One night something awoke Jenn and something was telling her to go in her sister's room, so she did. As she walked in, there was that scum ball, and he was TRYING to sexually abuse Jodi, but Jenn did not let that happen. Jenn walked in the room and started hitting Robbie. Even though she had EB she was a strong little girl! This means that, in the end, the sexual abuse, mental abuse and physical abuse went on for years to come, so life was not getting any better!! The kids had been happy after Gary went to jail, and so was Joanne, but when she met Robbie she was a totally different person.

Time went on and they lost that nice trailer they had because Joanne would not pay the rent. Robbie was still with Joanne, and living with them.

Jennifer didn't realize she had a disability at this time because so much was going on in her life, but soon it would become all too real. Jennifer's health was deteriorating; she would get an infection every month and would be in the hospital for a week. Jennifer was suffering from malnutrition because her mother was not caring for her the way Joanne should have been.

Jennifer weighed 42 lbs. and was 4 feet tall; this was very bad. Jenn was nothing but skin and bones; she almost died a few times because the infections were so bad. The hospital was like a second home for Jennifer. She liked the hospital better than her home, she was so happy when she would go in because she was away from the bad life she did not want. Jennifer learned to block the past as a defense mechanism, so in turn she did not remember much; there is much more to the story she does not want to reveal and has blocked out.

Jennifer was very depressed because of the life her brother and sister had. She would think of killing herself and what would be the best way to do it. She thought of this a lot. She thought of not telling anyone about one of the infections and then just let it get so bad where nobody could do anything to get it better, but there was something that would stop her from doing this, and that was her love for her brother and sister. She wanted to be there for them. Jennifer was particularly close to Jodi, she saw what Jodi had to go through and Jenn felt her sister's pain! Jenn's brother, however, never got in trouble and rarely got hit, although Jenn remembers when Joanne got so mad one time that she went and ripped the phone cord out of the wall and started to beat him with it! Jodi and Anthony where very close too; Jennifer, however, was not that close to her brother.

Even as an adult it hurt Jennifer a lot to simply think of what her and her siblings went through. Despite the rough childhood and EB, Jennifer was a very happy girl. She taught a lot of people a lot of things and not to take things for granted!!

In the end, Jodi and Jennifer went to live with Grammy and their Daddy.

Jennifer & Jodi's brother couldn't come because there was not enough room in the apartment that they had. Anthony went to live in a boys ranch; he needed to be there.

Jennifer wanted everyone to know that she enjoyed her life as best that EB would allow. She learned how to deal with EB and how to handle it with people in general. There are many different kinds of people out there, there are some rude people who do not understand about EB, and then there are very sweet and caring people. Jennifer had been told by many, but mostly by her Grandmother, that she was very unique and special. She tried hard to reach her goals in life, get her own place, get her own driver's license and more.

Sadly, Jennifer passed away on May 18th, 2005 due to kidney problems. She had been on dialysis. Jennifer graduated from Eau Gallie High School and attended B. C. C., where she was a member of the International Honor Society.

She was a member of Holy Name of Jesus Catholic Church and was a spokesperson for the Dystrophic Epidermolysis Bullosa Research Association (DebRA).

~

Living with Epidermolysis Bullosa

Our EB Story

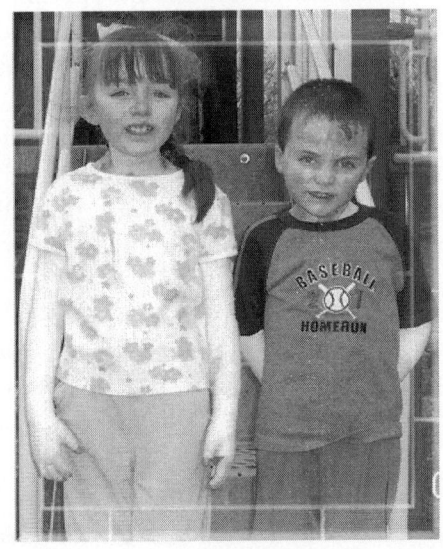

By Molly B.
ebkids@earthlink.net
Ohio, USA

Molly B. is the mother of 2 children with Recessive Dystrophic Epidermolysis Bullosa (RDEB). Her daughter Rachel is the oldest and is 8 years old. Her son Matthew is 6 years old. They live in Ohio, USA. Molly's story tells of the birth of her children and the struggles her and her husband went through shortly after each birth.

I was born and raised in Columbus, Ohio. I have two wonderful parents and two younger sisters. I have a bachelor's degree from Ohio State University.
I never thought of being a stay at home mom, I had always pictured myself as a career woman. But as many of you know things don't always go as we have planned.
On September 15, 1995 I married my high school sweetheart Greg and began thinking about having a family. Our first addition to our family was a white and red Cocker Spaniel we named Maggie. Then in January of 1997 I was feeling some changes in my body and began to suspect that I might be pregnant. I ended up taking a home pregnancy

test and it was positive. I was so excited; I had never wanted anything so much in my life. I had been helping take care of my 6-month old niece and I loved every minute of it.

I called the doctor and scheduled my first prenatal visit which would be another month away. Well, I didn't make it to that doctor's appointment. A couple weeks after I found out I was pregnant I ended up miscarrying. I was totally devastated! I had never felt so much pain in my life both physically and emotionally. My doctor couldn't give me any reason why this happened to me, but I now believe that this child would have probably been affected with Epidermolysis Bullosa (EB) had it lived. Somehow over time I began to slowly heal from this traumatic experience.

It wasn't until January 1998 that I found myself in a similar situation as the previous year. I again found out by a home pregnancy test that I was pregnant. This time I could not feel the joy about this pregnancy that I had felt the previous year. I was so nervous about having another miscarriage. This time I did make it to my first doctor's appointment and saw my baby's heartbeat on the ultrasound monitor. It was the most awesome feeling to know that a baby was growing inside of me.

This pregnancy went along wonderfully. I didn't have very many problems, besides being pregnant throughout the hottest part of the summer. This baby was due on September 17th. Almost a week overdue my doctor decided he would induce my labor. I had a very easy labor that only lasted about 10 hours. At 10:53pm on September 22nd my first child was born. We named her Rachel Nicole. She was a very large baby weighing 9 pounds and 21 inches long.

Everything was fine with Rachel until the nurse started cleaning her off; at that point the nurse noticed that Rachel's mouth was bleeding along with one of her fingers. She then pulled the vacuum suction off the wall and began suctioning out Rachel's mouth. This did not help at all, it only made things worse. Rachel was taken to the NICU in the hospital until the doctors and nurses could find out what was wrong with her.

It was within 24 hours that Rachel was diagnosed with a devastatingly painful skin disorder called Recessive Dystrophic Epidermolysis Bullosa (RDEB).

We had never heard of this before and didn't know what to expect for our daughter's future. I couldn't believe this was happening to us, first a miscarriage and now this terrible skin disorder. I kept thinking: "What have we done to deserve this?"

Rachel ended up staying in the NICU for 7 days. Those 7 days and the next 6 months were the hardest days of my life. Rachel's skin was very fragile and would blister or slough off from the slightest touch. We needed to wrap her like a mummy to protect her skin from damage and pop the blisters that she would get.

All we wanted was to be parents to a healthy newborn baby, but instead, we had to pretty much learn to be a nurse to our child.

After we got Rachel home her skin started to improve dramatically. The care and love we gave her helped her immensely. This is not to say that she didn't suffer terribly from the pain that EB caused her, because she did, but as each day went by we began to develop a routine for bathing and bandage changes that seemed to reduce the amount of pain that Rachel endured. Despite the fact that Rachel has EB, she manages to be a happy and healthy little girl.

Even though my daughter was born with this terrible disorder I absolutely LOVED being a mother. I never could have imagined what it was going to be like to be the mother and protector of this beautiful child. It was the most awesome feeling ever. I loved being a mother so much that I desperately wanted to have another child immediately. Everyone that I spoke to thought that I was crazy, but I couldn't help how I felt. It wasn't until Rachel was 15 months old that I finally convinced my husband, Greg, that we would be able to handle having another baby.

I found out I was pregnant on January 7th, 2000 by doing a home pregnancy test. I was so excited to be having another child. This time I had feelings of anxiousness due to the fact that this baby had a 25% chance of having EB like Rachel. I knew that there was this risk with having another baby, but I never really let myself believe that this baby might have EB also.

Everyone had always told me that God would never give anyone more than they could handle, and I really believed we had all we could handle caring for Rachel, but on April 10th, through an amniocentesis, we found out that the baby boy I was carrying would also be affected with EB.

I was devastated and felt like my world was crashing down around me. This was a really hard time for me because I thought there was no way I could care for two children with this awful disease. Another problem that I was having is that I was getting pressure from my husband to terminate the pregnancy. Even though I didn't want to bring another child into this world to endure a life of pain and suffering, I couldn't bring myself to terminate this pregnancy.

After several weeks of arguing and disagreeing, Greg and I finally decided that we would have this baby boy and give him the best quality of life we possibly could.

On August 28th, 2000 we went to the hospital to have my labor induced. At 5:23pm Matthew Alan entered this world. He weighed 7 pounds 15 ounces and was 19 inches long. This labor was just as easy as the first and only lasted 8 hours.

Matthew was born without skin on both of his feet from the ankle down. Even though Matthew's feet were a mess, everything else about this delivery was exactly how I dreamt bringing a baby into this world would be. He never left our sight for one minute at the hospital and, unlike Rachel; he came home with us the same day I left the hospital. We were the ones to take care of him because we were the experts having cared for Rachel for 2 years.

The next few months just sort of flew by and Matthew's feet improved tremendously. Getting accustomed to handling two kids with the disorder was very difficult and time consuming, but with Greg's help we managed to develop a routine and get things done in a very timely manner; as each day went by things got a little smoother and easier.

I am very fortunate to have such a wonderful husband and immediate family to help out with Rachel and Matthew whenever things get a little hectic. Our family has been our biggest support system and we can't thank them enough for everything they do to help out.

I can't think of anything that compares to the joy and fulfillment that I have received being Rachel and Matthew's mother. They mean the world to me and I hope that one day they will be able to enjoy life without the hindrance of EB.

~

Living with Epidermolysis Bullosa

Our Angel, Baby J

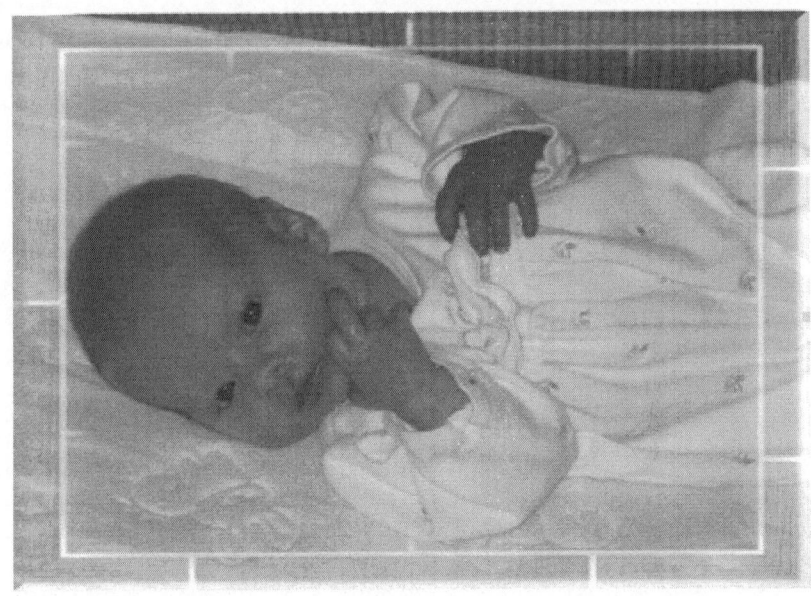

By Mandy Herreid
butterflymom1@msn.com
Idaho, USA

Mandy Herreid is mom to Jordan, a baby girl with Epidermolysis Bullosa, Junctional-Herlitz, who died when she was three months old. She and her husband, Dennis, also have a healthy five-year old daughter named Kate. Her story tells of her family's journey through Jordan's disease and what they have learned by experiencing her amazing life.

Our amazing family began the day Dennis and I were married on a beautiful June day in 1995. Almost seven years later, our first daughter, Kate Michelle, was born on February 28, 2002 by cesarean section because she was breech.

We wanted our children close in age, so we planned another pregnancy and were fortunate enough to have our girls 14 months apart. On April 26, 2003, our second daughter, Jordan Marie, was born in a repeat cesarean section.

The first thing I noticed was that a few of her fingernails were bright red. The nurses told me she was missing a few of them and assumed she had sucked them off in utero, which occurs occasionally.

In the recovery room, nurses noticed Jordan had a few small blisters on her bottom. They called our pediatrician, who called a dermatologist. The day after Jordan's birth, Dr. Mings came to see us in our hospital room. He told us he suspected a disease called Epidermolysis Bullosa. I specifically remember asking him the spelling and writing it down in a puzzle book I was working on.

That night, Dennis went home and looked EB up on the Internet. He called with the news that EB is not just another skin condition, and it could kill our baby girl. Before that moment, neither of us, nor our families, had any idea that a skin condition could be fatal. Throughout that second night of Jordan's life, I held on to my baby for all I was worth. I couldn't bear the thought that this beautiful gift from God may not be with us for very long.

No one in Boise, Idaho knows much about EB. We are thankful for this, since no one knew to tell me not to breastfeed my baby and no one tried to keep her in the hospital; we were sent home after two nights. Soon, Jordan had blisters everywhere that something sticky had been placed on her body during the hospital stay. We called the dermatologist with information from the Internet EB community. He then provided us with the supplies we needed to take care of Jordan's wounds.

In the beginning, Jordan did not seem to be in pain. She was a calm, gentle baby who loved to nurse and be entertained by her big sister. We reveled in the light of our precious baby for those first few weeks.

On May 13, 2003, Dennis' birthday, we got the biopsy-confirmed diagnosis that our Baby J had Junctional Epidermolysis Bullosa. Of course, we didn't know the type at that point, and we prayed she had non-Herlitz. At the same time, Jordan's pain was beginning to be evident, and we felt selfish at our thoughts of wanting her alive and with us in that kind of pain.

Wound dressing changes were excruciating for Jordan and moving around opened painful blisters on her ears and around her mouth. We stopped breastfeeding, so she wouldn't have to expend the energy and put her on a condensed formula. We spent countless, heartbreaking hours lancing, cleaning, and dressing her many blisters. During those times, we were so grateful to have our family and friends with us to help. Many people came over for hours at a time to watch Kate or help me give Jordan a bath. Caring for a baby with EB is not something a parent can do alone, and we were so blessed to have people so willing to sacrifice for our family.

In June, Baby J's cry became hoarse. While my mom stayed with Kate, we took Jordan to Seattle to see EB specialists. They were unable to tell us if she had Junctional-Herlitz, but Dennis and I both felt they suspected it. We talked about the possibilities available for feeding and breathing if the blisters were affecting her esophagus and trachea to the point she could not eat or breathe. Both Dennis and I felt these measures were unfair to our baby and may serve only to prolong her suffering; we only hoped we would never have to make those decisions.

God had a different plan for our family than what we thought we wanted. Toward the end of July, Jordan stopped eating. Her breathing changed, and her color turned bluish-gray. We started her on morphine and held her constantly, knowing she would be free of pain soon. On July 30, 2003, after having lived 95 days on this earth, Jordan died in her Daddy's arms. Almost all of our family was there with us when Jordan passed away. We spent time holding her and singing to her. Since she was no longer in pain, it was much easier to hold her without worrying about hurting her fragile, little body.

Two weeks later, while Dennis and I stood on a balcony overlooking the beach, he mentioned that he couldn't feel Jordan's presence and wished she would send him a shooting star, so that he would know she was all right. Almost immediately, a star shot across the sky. We watched two more shooting stars that night. Never in my life have I been surer that God exists and that he is watching over our precious Jordan.

Baby J's life was a beautiful time in our lives. We learned so much about our marriage and ourselves, and we discovered how very much our family and friends love us. Dennis and I felt the strength of God in ways we had never felt before; beyond that, we were given an angel for a child, and we are honored to be her family. We miss her so terribly, but we also know how happy she is in heaven with her perfect skin, able to run and play and enjoy being a child of God.

Since Jordan's death, her presence in our family has been constant. Kate talks about her almost daily. In our prayers, we ask God to kiss Baby J for us and let her know we miss her. Her perseverance and smile are our motivation.
It is our hope that Jordan continues to inspire and motivate people who were touched by her amazing life.

~

Living with Epidermolysis Bullosa

Mommy, Why Do I Always Have Blisters?

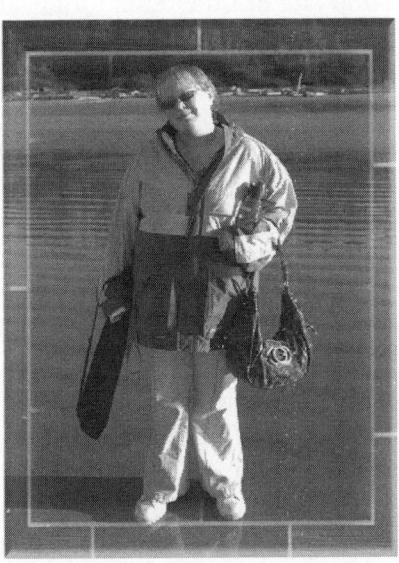

By Krystal A.
KrystalA1987@hotmail.com
British Columbia, Canada

Krystal A. is young woman who has EB Simplex Webber Cockayne disease. She has gone through a lot because of it, from being teased by other kids, to being fired from a hotel. She has also gotten a lot of information to try and help herself.

I was born on October 9th 1987 in Nanaimo, British Columbia. Approximately 24 months later, during the summer, my mum got the scare of her life. She woke up to see that her baby girl was one giant blister. Terrified, my mom rushed to the hospital where I was monitored for 2 days, and doctors could not explain why this was happening. And so it all began.

From this moment on my mother Fiona did whatever she could to try and help. She took me to specialist after specialist to find out why I kept getting all these blisters, but no one knew. Some doctors said to pop the blisters if they were bothersome. Some doctors said not to pop them. Every doctor said to soak my feet in Epsom Salts. So that's what my mum did. She popped the blisters for me while I was too young to do it myself. I remember how much they used to hurt in the bathroom, after being popped with a sterile needle. The air would hit the open wound, and would sting like nothing else. Quite often they would bring me to tears. My mum would then cover them with polysporin and a bandage to prevent infection.

My mum always did the best she could do for me. I remember one summer we were living in Courtney, BC., and I went to show her a big blister that I thought was cool. It was on my ankle and was shaped like a twister. My mum rushed me into the bathroom, sterilized a sewing needle and popped it. I remembered not understanding why she was popping my blister. It wasn't hurting and it was cool looking. I now understand, knowing more about EB that it was the best thing she could do for me.

My mum would always make me feel better when they were hurting, which was almost daily. She and my stepdad (who I have always considered being my only dad, and therefore will just refer to him as my dad) would always play games with me indoors since I couldn't do much outside. They would color with me, play board games, and video games, and just about anything else I wanted.

When I would go to school I would always feel left out. I couldn't run and play like everyone else. My feet would hurt really badly, and they always made you go outdoors on recess and lunches, unless it was raining. I did poorly in gym, because of the pain, and had no doctor's note to excuse me from it, or even part of it due to my feet. A lot of kids made fun of me because I could not participate in gym very much, and didn't do too well, although when we would play floor hockey or soccer I would always be the goalie since that was all I could do. I became so good that the kids would always want me to be their goalie.

Then I reached grade eight, my first year of high school. We would always do a 20-minute run each day at the beginning of class, and then we would get into the rest. That's where a lot of the problems started. Between gym class and walking between all the classes, at the end of the day I couldn't even walk. There were even times that I would have to crawl around the house.

My mum wrote me notes to take to my Gym teacher so I would only have to work for half of the hour and 20 minute class. My Gym teacher was not very accepting of it, and was trying to make me do more. Then one day I pulled off my shoes and socks, and showed him the better of the two feet. He took one quick look then turned away real quick, and he looked almost as if he was going to cry. Since then he never bothered me about how much I participated in Gym, as long as I tried.

While everything was going on with my Gym teacher, my mum took me to the family doctor, who yet again sent me to a specialist to see if there were any new developments. This time I got to see a fantastic dermatologist by the name of Dr. Hankock. He was the 13th and final specialist that I have had to see. He was able to diagnose me in August 2001 with Epidermolysis Bullosa Simplex. Finally some answers!

Dr. Hankock was absolutely terrific. He even got out his big text books and went through a lot of information with me. We also found out that the ridges on my brittle fingernails were linked to it. Thankfully he also gave me a note to take to school to take me out of Gym class altogether as walking the halls from class to class was more than enough already.

I still remember the relief that came over me that day. Finally we know why I kept getting all those horrible blisters. We found out that, yes, I need to be popping them, and taking extra care of them. He also gave me advice on how to prevent the blisters. However, we had nothing to help with the pain.

One day I was in my local Wal-Mart with my mom; we found some foot creams with mint, peppermint, and balm mint in them, so my mum bought me some to try.

Wow! The foot creams made such a huge difference!

From then on I started putting the mint foot lotion on my feet in the morning before school. I would put it on when I got home and my feet were the worst. Then before bed I would go through the torture of popping my own blisters in the bathroom and putting the polysporin and bandages on. To help with the stinging, I would also put the mint lotion on, never on the open wound though. I would put it around the blisters, which soothed my skin and helped reduce the stinging.

At the age of 15 I got my first job, working in a Chinese fast food place, and that's when I really learned how bad EB can be, especially when I moved on to later jobs. I wanted to be a hotel manager, and learnt that you have to work your way up from the bottom, being housekeeping. I worked there for about two weeks before I ended up having to tell them about it because I couldn't walk fast enough from the pain of the blisters and therefore couldn't clean the rooms fast enough. They fired me that day because of it, but still wanted me to come in for my Saturday shift because it would be really busy.

Needless to say I said no.

One summer I went onto my favorite search engine and typed in Epidermolysis Bullosa, and it came up with www.debra.org. I went through the site, and learned even more of what I had, and what other conditions that I have been effected with that I didn't even think could be related. It's amazing how much it really can affect you without you even knowing it. I also learned that there are many different sub-types of EB, and all about EB Simplex. I learned that the version of EB Simplex that I have is called "Webber Cockayne". I also learned that the ulcer that I had in my eye, and the pain in my eyes that I have had for years, are also related to the EB. My Optometrist couldn't figure out why they would be related, but they are, since the cells that our eyes are made of are the same that our skin is made of.

I am also very happy to see that there are many new studies being conducted to help all of us suffering from all types of EB. I just ordered online a hoodie from Debra.Org to go towards the research, and awareness of EB.

I really hope that the studies are successful to bringing relief to all of us who have been diagnosed, and will be diagnosed in the future with EB. I know how horrible it has been for me and the pain I have suffered with my "mild" form of EB. I can only imagine how those with worse cases feel, and my heart goes out to you all.
Always stay strong, we are in this together.

~

Living with Epidermolysis Bullosa

Xander's Story

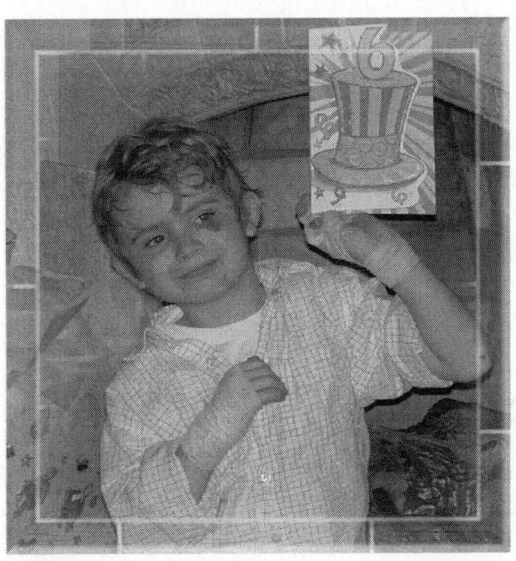

By Venus S.
bvandx@kc.rr.com
Missouri, USA

Venus S. is the mother of Xander, a six year old child with Junctional EB. They live in Kansas City, Missouri (USA). This is Venus' only child since she and her husband made the decision not to have subsequent children after Xander was born. Her story highlights the birthing and newborn experience she had with Xander.

Xander was conceived in Norway on our honeymoon. Brad and I were hoping to conceive a child within our first year of marriage, but never expected it to happen so fast. When I was about six weeks pregnant I began cramping and spotting blood. The OB asked me to come into the office for a sonogram to check the baby. Xander's heartbeat was already audible and everything appeared to be normal. The spotting ceased.

I was very nauseous for most of my pregnancy and lost weight in the first few months. By the second trimester things seemed to calm down. I started gaining weight nicely and enjoyed the feeling of the growing life inside of me.

I remember Xander being very active in utero. I would often remark to Brad about how busy Xander had been during the day only for him to continue being very active throughout the night. After weeks of poor sleep I finally took some Tylenol PM to help me sleep as my little boy moved restlessly inside of me. I knew he was very active, but didn't address the situation with my OB because my friends reassured me that it was just a good sign that he was healthy. The likely reality of why he was so restless haunts me.

My membranes ruptured two weeks before my due date as I sat in bed watching the news with Brad. I sat up most of the night feeling pretty good experiencing what I would best describe as menstrual cramps. After very little rest, I began the morning by engaging in a large breakfast and went for a walk around the neighborhood with a friend. By lunchtime we decided that we had better prepare to go to the hospital, but first I had a nice lunch. Once at the hospital it was quickly confirmed that my membranes had indeed ruptured. (To this day, I believe it was one of Xander's long, thick fingernails that tore my membrane.) Unfortunately, I didn't progress much once I got to the hospital and the hardest part of the journey lay ahead. I was determined not to have any medication, so I worked on my breathing and enlisted the help of a birthing ball and Jacuzzi tub to ease my lower back pains. Eventually I gave in to exhaustion and received an Epidural!

After 39 hours it was finally time to deliver Xander! In spite of the long labor, the delivery only took 20-25 minutes.

The first clue that something might be wrong was a visible blister on the crown of Xander's head. His head would appear, but because I was so tired and couldn't push hard enough he would disappear back inside of me again only to partially reappear a few moments later when I got the strength to push again. I remember everyone telling me to touch his head so I could get a better idea of how close he was to being born, but I didn't want to touch him. Perhaps it was a mother's instinct that told me I shouldn't. When Xander was finally completely delivered the doctor put him on my abdomen as I had requested, but before I could even lift my head to see him, the nurses had taken him away.

I never saw him directly following birth. Instead, I saw about 15 people rush into the room and begin to work on Xander. His Apgar score was only 2 at birth. Once they got him breathing he received an 8. They rushed him out of the delivery room very quickly and I was left to deliver a placenta that didn't want to detach.

The very first time I saw my baby, a few hours later, he was in the highest level NICU nursery already bandaged on his arms and legs with IV's running into his belly. They let me hold him for a few minutes as I cried.

Xander was born missing about 50 percent of the skin on his little body. His hands and feet were completely raw with many other large raw areas along his arms, legs, and other areas. Fortunately for us, there was a Neonatologist on duty who had seen a baby born with Epidermolysis Bullosa (EB) earlier in her career. Also, a dermatologist was present who had studied under a doctor who specialized in doing skin grafts for children with EB. I heard what the doctor said when he told me what he thought was wrong with Xander's skin, but I certainly didn't understand it.

The dermatologist ordered an electron microscopy test to substantiate that Xander had EB. The results confirmed EB and seemed to indicate that it might be the Junctional subtype. We then forwarded a skin biopsy to Dr. Fine in North Carolina for confirmation. The first biopsy was not performed correctly so the results were inconclusive. The second skin biopsy led to the diagnosis of Junctional non Herlitz EB. This is an autosomal recessive genetic disorder.

Specific information about the different subtypes of EB is available on the ebinfoworld.com website.

With everything we have learned about EB we feel that there are still just as many questions. We have no family history of EB. Fortunately, Xander continues to do very well. The most regularly affected areas continue to be his hands, feet, mouth, head, nose, and anus. He has blistered in virtually every part of his body at one time or another. When Xander was a baby he was eating formula almost exclusively with the assistance of a special bottle. We tried to get him to eat regular baby food, but he refused it most of the time. We are fortunate that his weight is very good and he is extremely happy in spite of the constant discomfort he experiences.

Before Brad and I could leave the hospital with Xander we were both pseudo-certified as able to manage his wound care. Once we got home the daily grind began. It was a constant search for new blistering that we could lance and prevent from becoming huge puss filled masses that would encompass an entire hand or foot. We couldn't bathe Xander due to the pain he would experience from water on his open wounds, so we began sponge bathing him the best we could. He also lost all of the skin on his bottom and abdomen, so diapering was very challenging.

I had dreamed about how wonderful the breast-feeding experience would be, but this was impossible since Xander blistered badly in his mouth. Instead we fought to find creative ways to get food in him without him having to suck. We tried everything from dropping milk into his mouth with a syringe, to using a special nipple for babies with a cleft palate, to orthopedic nipples that we could cut a larger hole into and apply Vaseline around the base. Xander used a special Mead Johnson bottle that we could squeeze so that Xander didn't have to suck as hard.

One of the most important things I have learned is how important nutrition is to children with EB. We give Xander a protein powder supplement, adult liquid Centrum, and an oral zinc supplement to help replace what he loses through the open wounds.

Having a newborn is difficult for parents. Having a newborn whose skin blisters or tears due to friction, heat, or humidity is maddening. We questioned daily whether or not Xander could do certain things that most parents take for granted like riding in a car seat, sitting in a swing, and wearing onesies. Every time we experimented with things we were left to wait and see the consequences.

After Xander was a few months old we became comfortable enough to venture out to a store with him. We then had to endure the barrage of questions from shoppers. We have seen people begin to approach us only to then scrunch up their face awkwardly and quickly turn away once they see that something is wrong with our son. People have commented that he must scratch himself a lot, or think that he has chicken pox, or simply not know what to think. Most of the time, people just don't get it! They don't understand how pervasive and permanent this is. They make silly attempts to compare what Xander is living with to relatively minor conditions. Many people simply cannot accept that he will not outgrow this and that most children with this condition do not live a normal life span.

When Xander was a newborn, I didn't know if he would live to see his first birthday. Now, I know that he will likely see many more. I have also learned that he can and will do far more than I ever imagined. There will also be much physically that he cannot do. The fact remains; he is a tremendous little spirit and an inspiration to his parents, family, and friends!

Like Mother ~ Like Son

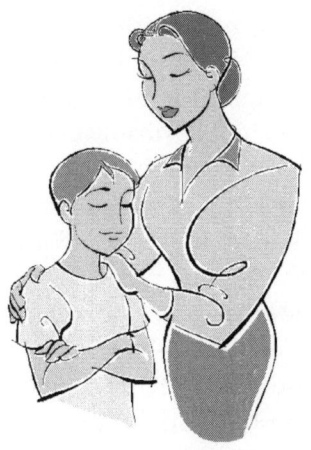

By Carol M.
cameo.anew@gmail.com
California, USA

Carol M. is a 66-year-old woman with EB Simplex who also has a 45-year-old son with EBS. She lives in California and her son and his family live in Provo, UT. She also has a 42-year-old daughter with no signs of EB. When she was a child she was treated free of charge by two dermatologists who were studying EB and felt she was helping them as much or more than they were helping her.

My name is Carol and I was born 66 years ago (1941) with Epidermolysis Bullosa Simplex. I am not exactly sure just when my parents first noticed the problem, but I do know that our family doctor told them at that time that, as far as he knew, there was nothing that could be done. I do not know if he was aware of the diagnosis or not. I have one brother who is 18 months older and he did not have any signs of EB. He is married and has four children and none of his children have any signs of any form of EB.

Throughout my father's life, he had very sensitive skin that did tear very easily (we called him "knuckle-nicker") and he would get blisters on his feet when he wore his "switchman's" boots without wearing the proper heavy socks (during his early career with Southern Pacific

Railroad he was a switchman).

His sister also told me that their mother had also had some similar type problems with her feet, but I have no first had knowledge of this.

My father was promoted to a junior officer for Southern Pacific and transferred to California from Oregon when I was only three years old. At that time, their doctor told them that they should not take me from one doctor to another looking for an answer because they might find an unscrupulous doctor who would promise to find a cure, only to give them false hope, and take their money.

I can remember my parents saying that when we lived in Oregon, or when we would go back to visit, we would go out on my Uncle's boat and they would watch the blisters pop up on my feet. They also would tell me stories of my maternal grandmother hardly being able to stand being in the same house if my mother was taking care of my blisters.

When I was in the 3rd grade my teacher's husband was a podiatrist. Although EBS was not in his field, he was very interested because my blisters affected primarily my feet. Also, we lived in the very small East Bay community of San Lorenzo Village and teachers took much more interest in their students back then. My teacher's husband, Dr. Nelson, referred me to a dermatologist who worked in the same building with him.

Two dermatologists worked in practice together, Dr. Lincoln and Dr. Nordstrom. They were treating at least one other EB patient that we were aware of and were glad to take me as a patient without charging my parents, as they felt they were learning and gaining as much or more than we were.

These Doctors took the water out of some blisters, the skin off of some, and even removed one whole blister off the top of my left foot. I can remember the doctor telling the nurse to handle that blister with care because it took me a long time to get one in just the right spot for him to be able to remove it.

At one point, they asked me to get as many blisters as I could so they could take pictures for medical books. I could not even get shoes on to go to school I had so many blisters. I was crawling around my house on my hands and knees.

They circled all 16 of the blisters on my feet with gentian violet so they would show up on film; so somewhere in ancient medical books are pictures of my blisters. They also took me to several Medical Conventions with them, the one I remember the most was at Letterman General Hospital at the Army Presidio in San Francisco. As I remember, they treated me for several years.

When I was expecting my first child in 1962, I went back to them and asked what the chances were that my children would have some form of EB and they told me they were "slim to none". In September of that year, my son Steve was born and when he got his first blisters on his hands from pulling himself up in his crib I took him back to them and told them: "Here is your slim to none chance." They did some testing of his blisters to make sure it was not something other than EB and when the results came back, they confirmed that he did indeed have EBS. Because of the way he crawled, he then started getting them on his elbows and knees as well.

After having lived with EBS for that many years, it was very difficult to think that now I was going to have to watch my son go through the same problems I had gone through. I made the mistake at that time of not asking for both my son's and my medical records. That was so many years ago I am sure all of our records are destroyed by now.

Our EBS seems to be limited mostly to our hands and feet and of course gets much worse in summer as the weather gets hotter. There have been a few exceptions to that rule of thumb, like when I got a blister on my rear-end when my stepdaughter took me bareback horseback riding; or when I had blisters up my shins when I went roller-skating with high top shoe skates.

Steve and I both consider ourselves very fortunate indeed, when we read stories of others who have much more serious cases of EB. As I got older, my parents tried very hard to let me make my own decisions about what I could and could not do because of my EBS and in turn, I did the same with Steve. We have always known what the consequences of the activities we wanted to participate in would be and if we wanted to do something bad enough we just would do whatever it is we wanted to do. We still do the same. We know there are others that are just not able to do that.

Last year we visited Steve in Utah and he took us to show us Capitol Reef. Of course, there are places you just cannot see without hiking in to see them, so we did just that. As usual, I did not stop soon enough and of course, you have to hike back out! After a day and a half of that, we were both walking on eggs for several days. The same thing happened when they came and we went to show them Yosemite. We do what we want to do and suffer the consequences and our spouses and families are just great about supporting us in these activities.

Steve has a sister who is 23 months younger and, thankfully, she has no signs of EB and neither do any of her 3 sons nor does her one grandson, so we hope the chain has been broken.

~

Living with Epidermolysis Bullosa

A Second Generation with EB

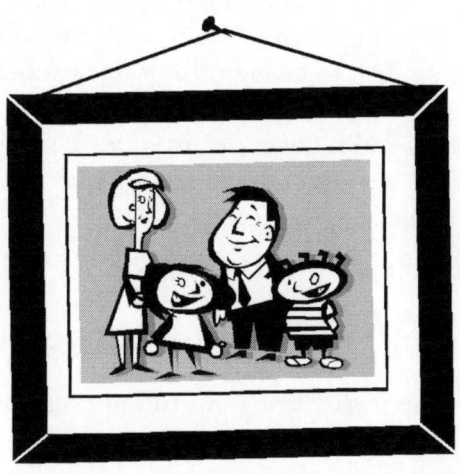

By Steve W.
steve.wygant@gmail.com
Utah, USA

Steve is a 45 year old father of two with EB Simplex. He is the second generation (following his mother Carol) with EB and has two children (who blessedly do not show signs of EB). He lives in Provo, Utah where he works for Brigham Young University.

Beginnings

My EB story actually starts before I was born. My mother has suffered with EB Simplex throughout her life and there is some evidence that her father also had some form of it.

When she found that she was pregnant with me she asked her doctors about the chances of her baby having EB. At that time (1962) knowledge of the genetic transfer was pretty weak; the doctor told her the chances were slim and none that I would have EB. Imagine her shock when I started pulling myself up on the side of the crib and blistered the palms of my hands. When I started to crawl, my hands and knees blistered as well, so I learned to crawl alternating between hands and elbows, whichever was less painful. She told me that I looked like an army man sneaking around on my belly.

My own earliest memories related to EB go back to when I was four or five and my mother would pop my blisters. I would lie on the couch with my feet in her lap while she sliced the blisters open with a razor blade and drained the fluid. I would scream, burying my head in a pillow to muffle the sound. Then she would carefully dress them and put soft socks on my feet to cushion the pain and help the open sores to heal.

During my childhood it never occurred to me that she had to endure the same thing when she was my age and that now she had to take care of my blisters in addition to her own.

~

Dealing with EB as a child: challenges and adjustments

Growing up with EB was no fun of course. I know now that having EB Simplex is a cakewalk compared to the more devastating strains, but I never realized this as a child. I just knew that I was different from my peers. I could not do all of the things they could do, or at least I couldn't do them for very long and if I did, there was a price to be paid. Running created blisters on my feet, and swinging a bat or a racket blistered my hands so most sports were out. Not wanting to be completely left out I played as much as I could, but that was usually not very much, and it is hard to get good at a sport that you can't practice.

My mother taught me that I should not let the blisters determine what I could do, but that I should do what I wanted to do, knowing what my limitations were, and accept that sometimes the consequences would be blistered hands or feet. While she was always sympathetic and took care of my blisters she never let me feel sorry for myself. This was just something that had to be dealt with.

Despite my mother's encouragement, it was almost inevitable that sports and physically active pursuits were not my thing. I recall marching in a parade once as a Cub Scout, just once though. Whatever the excitement was it must not have been worth the price I paid. I eventually learned to enjoy activities that were physically passive but more mentally engaging. Model airplane building became a passion. As a boy I had a great collection of model fighter and bomber airplanes from World War II. I can still recall how exciting it was when my uncle, who was in the Air Force in WWII came to visit and I could tell him about all of the planes hanging from my ceiling. I think I actually knew more about most of them than he did. I also got very good at jigsaw puzzles and learned to play chess well enough to be the school chess nerd. Most importantly I learned to love books. I read voraciously. I discovered Tolkein, Alistair MacLean, Louis La'Amour, and many others. I read books about animals, books about war, books about adventures in far-off places, perhaps experiencing vicariously some of the things I could not do or did not think I could do directly.

~

Change of scenery

One of the major turning points in my EB was a move we made when I was in the fourth grade. Up until that time we lived in the San Francisco Bay area, which has a fairly mild climate. However, from the fourth grade until I finished high school my family lived in Bakersfield, California, where summer temperatures range from lows in the 80s and 90s to highs over 100. Since heat makes the blistering worse this climate was particularly challenging. Walking to and from school was ok in the cooler months, but was a real problem towards the end of the school year. Fortunately the school year ended at about the same time the temperatures topped 100 for the first time.

Participating in Physical Education classes at school was often my biggest problem. My mother would write notes to excuse me when my feet were sore or I had blisters, or it was just too hot, but not too many male high school PE teachers are sympathetic to boys who can't participate. Peers were often worse. The gamut of reactions ran from disbelief ("Why don't you just wear thick socks?" or "Everyone gets a blister occasionally, what's your problem?") to taunting and ridicule. Of course they had no way of knowing that this was a real disease. Since I didn't look any different than anyone else (and didn't usually take my socks off to show blisters when I had them) it was hard for them to accept that there was anything really different about me.

Twice-yearly bouts with pneumonia during six years of early childhood had also stunted my growth, so I must have seemed like the perfect sissy-boy. It was probably not the case as often as I recall, but I remember being left out of games at recesses a lot and, of course, any time a choice for athletic teams had to be made I was the last one picked. Even the girls were picked before I was; talk about humiliation! Even when I could participate I didn't have much to offer the football, kickball, baseball or basketball teams so they mostly ignored me.

The theme of doing what I could and living with the consequences continued through adolescence; the most exciting (and painful) memory from high school was a 12-hour dance marathon I joined in with my future wife. After five hours I could hardly walk, but it was the most fun I had ever had and stopping was out of the question. After 12 hours I could only crawl away. I crawled around the house for two days until the blisters started to heal. When I was 19 I served a two-year mission for the Church I belong to. In some areas we had a car, but in others I had to walk or ride a bicycle. (I won't describe the problems, which came from riding a bike all day!)

~

Adulthood

As an adult I have tried to be active. While the blisters continue to be a hindrance I try not to let them stop me completely. Yard work is a challenge, a couple of hours mowing the lawn or digging in the garden and I am done, but it is worth the effort and pain. A few years ago I decided to take up golf so that I could be one of the guys and play occasionally with my father. The reality is that I haven't learned the game yet. It's tough to get the swing down right when practice is limited to a couple of hours once a week. Actually my dad tells me that the problems with my golf swing have less to do with blisters than the fact that I am just uncoordinated.

I have also taken up landscape photography as a hobby and part-time business. This is a wonderful creative outlet but most places I like to go to shoot pictures require some hiking to get to. While I feel very fortunate that I can walk enough to get to some of the beautiful places I have been able to photograph, I know that there are some places I would like to shoot that I never will.

Last summer my daughter and I went on a four-day, 60 mile canoeing trip with her best friend and her best friend's father. I prepared as well as I knew how by wearing bicycling gloves and bringing along all of the skin care gear I could, but after the first ten miles my hands were already blistered. Fortunately there was enough current that the river carried us without strenuous paddling for much of the trip, and some creative padding of my gloves and switching paddling from one side of the canoe to the other often allowed me to finish the trip. While it took several days for the blisters on my hands to heal it was a wonderful trip for Lyndsay and I, and I would do it again in a minute.

~

Lessons

Like many people with disabilities, it is a challenge for me to avoid letting EB define me. It is obviously true that there are things I would like to do be able to do that I can't. There are things that I would like to have been able to do at many periods of life that has not been possible. However, I cannot think that I am a victim of this condition, and I have never thought of myself as being disabled.

I have learned to accept the limitations and deal with them as effectively as possible, even when that means swallowing some ego. Several years ago we took a family vacation to Disneyland. Throughout the first day I walked wherever I wanted to. However, by the second day I was blistered so badly that I could not walk. Over my objections, my wife obtained a wheelchair for me, which I reluctantly agreed to use. I felt awkward and self-conscious about using the wheelchair because I could walk when I needed to badly enough, but I certainly could not have enjoyed the day with my family if I had insisted on trying to walk through the park. Similarly, I finally swallowed my pride this year and obtained a handicapped-parking badge for my car. I hope to never use it, but if I need to at some point I can.

I guess that sums up how I see myself in relation to EB. It isn't me, but it does make me more aware of choosing what I do and where I put my time and effort. I am aware of the cost to me and to my family of the things I choose to do (and not to do). My true hope is that somehow I can find a way to help others with this condition that are worse off than I am to enjoy a better life.

~

Living with Epidermolysis Bullosa

Everlasting Butterfly

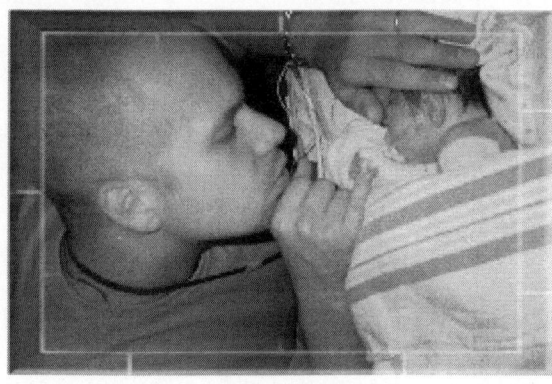

By Troy Medeiros
tmedeiros@everlastingbutterfly.com
Massachusetts, USA

Troy Medeiros is the father of Ava Elizabeth, who passed away at four months due to Junctional Epidermolysis Bullosa with Pyloric Atresia. Troy lives with his wife and three healthy daughters in Massachusetts, USA. His story characterizes the struggles with the pregnancy, birth, life, and death of his 2nd daughter. It also briefly explains the process that he and his wife went through that allowed them to have healthy twin girls after Ava.

In order to have a good understanding of the journey we went through, it is important to tell you a little bit about my family. My wife, Melanie, and I have been married since October of 1998, at which time she was pregnant with our first daughter, McKenzie Rae. I also have a son, Devin Michael, from a previous relationship. Both children are considered very healthy. McKenzie, in particular, was and is extremely lucky that she was able to dodge the bullet from this game of EB roulette that we were not even aware we played.

During my wife's pregnancy with Ava, McKenzie was very excited about being a big sister for the first time. Devin already had another little sister at home, so McKenzie was going through it for the first time. Nevertheless, they both really loved babies.

On June 16th, at approximately 10:00 pm, my wife had experienced some bleeding. We woke McKenzie up and rushed to the emergency room at Holy Family Hospital in Methuen, MA. Along with the bleeding, Melanie began contracting. At the time, we were not very concerned with the preterm labor because Melanie had experienced the same thing with McKenzie; who went full term. The doctors performed some ultrasounds, stress tests, and monitored the contractions throughout the night. The doctors could not control the contractions, so they transferred Melanie to St. Elizabeth's Hospital in Brighton, MA.

Severity unknown, we felt it was only a matter of time until the contractions would be under control and we would be home again. This could not have been further from the truth. Melanie lived at St. Elizabeth's for the next four weeks; she received many tests and was monitored constantly. Melanie was experiencing many emotions, mainly due to being away from her home and family.

It was a juggling experience with my work, my daughter, and visiting my wife, but, with our family's help, we were able to manage. I cannot even imagine what she went through and, on top of that, to find out it was only the beginning.

Melanie was anemic which, unknown at the time, is common with EB. Through ultrasound, the doctors noticed that Ava's stomach was enlarged and the amniotic fluid had some foreign matter in it. The doctors were not sure if it was bile or blood.

On July 13th, Melanie had an amniocentesis. The main reason was to relieve the pressure from excessive fluid but, also, to visually confirm the foreign matter. Healthy fluid is normally the color of apple juice, but my wife's fluid was a dark, greenish brown. It was immediately diagnosed as bile.

Again, this is common with Ava's rare type of EB and, as you read on, you will fully understand why. I remember asking the doctor if she had seen this before. She answered, yes, with confidence, to make sure we did not panic. The problem was that when we asked her how many times she had seen this, she answered only 'about five'. Not a very high number for someone with over twenty-five years of experience. So, safe to say, we were very concerned. By performing the amnio, we knew there was a risk of going into labor. It was not a surprise to receive a phone call, the next morning, explaining to me that Melanie needed to have an emergency C-section.

I immediately left work and headed to the hospital, which was in the outskirts of Boston. It was rush hour, so the traffic was stop and go, and I was extremely nervous I was not going to get there in time. Melanie called me numerous times to check where I was and I was tempted to call the police to see if I could get a police escort. Either way, I made it there just in time. Melanie was in the operating room; so I got into my scrubs as fast as I could and headed in. The doctors had already begun, but Ava was still playing hide and seek. Melanie was feeling very loopy and nauseous due to the anesthesia and

I felt helpless because all I could do was hold her hand and play with her hair.

What seemed like hours were only minutes before I saw my butterfly for the first time. The surgical wall that was placed on Melanie's chest prevented my wife from being able to see Ava. She asked me over and over if Ava was okay. I told her "Yes", and pretended to be happy, but what I saw had me scared to death.

Due to Melanie's current medical condition and her epilepsy, I knew I could not show the fear I felt and just told her Ava was perfect.

Ava was born at 9:24 am, on July 14, 2004, without skin on her right elbow or her stomach. I was in complete shock inside, but you would have thought I was an accomplished actor on that day. The nurses wrapped Ava up and brought her over so Melanie could see her and, with the blanket covering her, she looked as healthy as could be. Little did we know including the doctors, what was in store for us.

They immediately took Ava away, for what we thought, were the normal newborn tests. Even though I had seen Ava's wounds, I never imagined the severity. Once Melanie was back in her room, the doctors filled us both in about the best interest is to have her immediately transported to Children's Hospital in Boston. I was able to see and hold Ava before she left and, around 11:00 am, watched the medical team take her away in an incubator.

I went over to Children's Hospital the same day and met with the doctors. Melanie had to stay in the hospital for at least another three or four days, so the doctors set it up for her to be transferred to Brigham and Women's Hospital, which is connected to Children's Hospital. Unfortunately, my wife was not transferred for almost 36 hours later and she was emotionally and physically exhausted. After analyzing Ava's wounds and some preliminary tests, the doctors felt Ava had Epidermolysis Bullosa, but would not be sure without further testing.

EB has many forms and categorizations, so the severity of Ava's condition was still unknown. When I asked the doctor if people are able to live with this disease, he stated, yes, but, there were lethal forms as well, and it was too early to tell for sure which type Ava had. Genetic testing would need to be performed which could take six to eight weeks. What the doctors found through x-rays did help them to minimize the possible types. The doctors noticed Ava's stomach and small intestine were not connected (Pyloric Atresia); which was the cause of the bile in the amniotic fluid. Ava's form of EB was determined to be Junctional Epidermolysis Bullosa with Pyloric Atresia (JEB-PA), which is a recessive form. This meant that Melanie and I were both carriers of the gene mutation. Ava was vomiting whatever she swallowed because there was nowhere for it to go. This needed to be corrected and, two days after birth, Ava went in for surgery.

Although this was an emergency surgery, there was a lot of prep work that went into it. The surgeons were very concerned with Ava's skin and needed to determine how they were going to perform the procedure without creating more trauma. I remember getting together with the surgeon, anesthesiologist, and the rest of the medical staff right before the surgery. I was trying to be strong in front of my wife and daughter, but there was nothing I could do to hold back the tears. I feared that it was too much for this four-pound infant to handle and that I would never see her again. Ava showed everyone that she was a fighter and would not go down without swinging.

The surgery was a success and we felt Ava had a good chance of overcoming this disease. Of course, we began researching EB on the Internet and everything we were learning was decreasing our hopes. Now, do not get me wrong. We always kept faith and hoped our daughter would eventually come home. The problem was that Ava had one of the lethal forms of EB. Through all our research, we were only able to find one case of JEB-PA where the child lived to be a few years old. Not a very comforting find for a parent. EB is estimated to effect 1 in every 50,000 live births and Ava's form of the disease is estimated at 1 in 4 million; as if it was not rare enough.

Ava did seem to gradually improve over the first month and we were gaining hope. Since EB is a skin disease, we seemed to judge how well she was doing by the appearance of her skin. The problem was what the disease was actually doing to her internally. She had lesions in her mouth, esophagus, stomach, and intestines that were evident from the continuous blood loss. She suffered Tachycardia, fevers, blood clots, and seizures. She was never able to eat orally and actually did not reach her birth weight until she was about two months old. Her nutrition was provided through a central line that was inserted through her right thigh, traveled along the spine, and connected to a main artery by the heart. Ava also endured over fifty IV's that needed to be replaced because they would clot or come loose because they could not be sufficiently secured to her skin.

Putting my daughter's life into words is more difficult than I had thought. I do not feel there are the right words for someone to understand what we lived without actually living it for themselves. Imagine being afraid to hold your child because you will, not might, HURT them. Or, imagine watching your child suffer from the pain caused by lesions inside and outside his/her body, or from the sloughing of their inner tissues that were present in each and every stool. Imagine your child violently gagging on its own saliva because he/she cannot swallow. Envision how many medical procedures, test, or treatments involve doing something to the skin. How many of them require tape and the outcome when the bond of tape to skin is stronger than skin to patient!

I'm sure the seizures were not the most comforting, either. I think you probably get the picture.

Imagine bringing a child into this world and four months later guiding it into taking its last breath. I wish all I had to do was imagine, but I can't. I lived it and continue to live it every day of my life. Everyday decisions seem so minute when you are forced to make decisions on a person's life, especially your own child's. We had the greatest support from the hospital staff, family, and friends, which allowed us to feel confident that we made the right decisions. There was also the fear and guilt you feel while making those decisions. Are we just avoiding the inevitable, which, in turn, is prolonging her suffering? Or, could she be the one that finally survives and we cut her life short? No child should ever have to endure the pain this disease causes.

As horrible as it sounds, I consider my daughter lucky. She had to suffer what felt like forever in four months, but other forms allow years of physical and emotional pain.

Ava passed away in my wife's arms on November 20, 2004. Through the four months of Ava's life, I learned how much I hated this disease that most people do not even know exists. Never mind the fact that there is not a cure or even any treatment. It is, more or less, viewed as the outcome will be the outcome, so focus on the quality of life. We feel that we have done that for our daughter. Although her quality of life was not very good, it was all that EB would allow us to give her.

Since Ava, we have created a memorial website called Everlasting Butterfly (www.EverlastingButterfly.com), it has continued to expand into sources of EB information, EB events, support, and more. Ava's story is also told through a daily on-line journal that was kept throughout her life, which can be accessed through the site.

My wife and I know the reason we had Ava was because we wanted to expand our family. This experience did not take away that feeling, but minimized our options. Since we are both carriers of the gene mutation, we knew we had a 1 in4 chance with every pregnancy of reliving Ava's fate; a risk much too high to take and neither of us believed in abortion. So, we looked into a procedure called PGD (Pre-implantation Genetic Diagnosis) and IVF (In-Vitro Fertilization). In short, the doctors fertilize the woman's eggs and extract a single cell from each embryo, which is tested for the specific gene mutation.

In turn, each embryo is categorized as affected, carrier, or unaffected. Preferably, an unaffected embryo would be implanted, but the maturity of the embryo plays a part, so a carrier may still be used. After two attempts of this procedure, we now have healthy twin girls, one of which is a carrier. Since PGD has only been around for roughly ten years, we were informed we are believed to be the first documented, successful case of JEB-PA in the world!

This disease may have taken my daughter, but it has provided me with the inspiration to make EB known. Through books, charity events, media, anything and everywhere, we need to create awareness of EB. Awareness is the key to support; which is the key to finding a CURE!

On Earth, children with EB are known as Butterfly Children because their skin is as fragile as a butterfly's wings. Ava, and all EB Angels, are Everlasting Butterflies!

~

Jonathan's Story

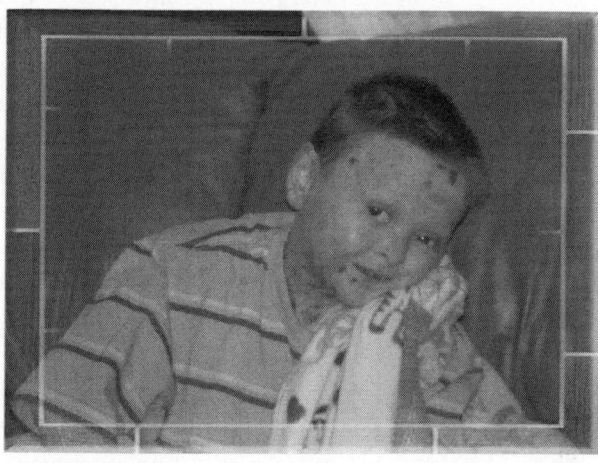

By Brenda G.
ebmommie@cox.net
www.ebzone.bravehost.com
Connecticut, USA

Brenda is the mother of Jonathan, an eight year old child with Recessive Dystrophic EB. Her story is about the birth of her son and how EB has affected her life. She also has a 10 year old daughter Ashley. Ashley does not have EB.

Jonathan was born in May 1999. We were so excited to be having another child that it never crossed our minds that there would be anything wrong with our new baby. All previous tests taken during the pregnancy came back fine; the pregnancy went well with no complications. Unfortunately they do not test for rare disorders when you are pregnant.

As with my daughter Ashley, I was now 2 weeks late, so we went into the hospital to get induced. The inductions moved along very quickly and within only a few short hours the moment came. We really thought we were going to have another girl so it was a shock when the doctor said: "It's a Boy."

We were so excited until the moment came when they started asking a lot of questions like: "Do you have herpes?" I kept saying no to all of their inquiries. All the nurses and doctors were huddled around my new baby and I was getting very nervous. I yelled out: "What's wrong with my baby", but all I got was that they were just checking him out. The nurses and doctors said that the cord was around his neck and he was a little blue. My husband said he looked fine but he had some small area with no skin, like his lips and one small place on his back. We thought it might be just because he was 2 weeks late and his skin was dry.

The nurses took Jonathan away after I got to hold him for what seemed to be one very short second; still not knowing or feeling there was anything wrong. A few hours later they allowed us to go see him in the neonatal ICU. Jonathan was under the warmer and to us he looked very good; his color was so much better, and from what we could see, his skin was beautiful. The nurses told us that when they pricked his heel to take blood for a test the skin just came off so they were going to have the doctors take a good look at him. Even so, we still did not think there was anything to wrong he looked so beautiful and healthy to us.

It was the middle of the night, so we went back to the room to rest, but we were a little worried. Not long after that a doctor came in and told us she thought Jonathan might have Epidermolysis Bullosa. I could not even pronounce it, never mind I had any clue what is was; the Doctor said it was a skin disorder, which included blistering but not much more, so now we started to panic.

I made a few phone calls to let family know we had a boy, but I didn't say too much else until we knew more; I simply did not want to worry anyone. The next time we were able to see our baby he was in an incubator; my heart just sank, I didn't hear a word the doctor said. I just looked at my little baby and cried; I just wanted to hold him and kiss him but they would not let me. The nurses told me not to worry, that they were not concerned I would get something from him but that he would get something from us, hence, as a precaution, they put Jonathan in the incubator with alert signs on it.

At this point the Doctor asked us if it would be ok to transfer the baby to another hospital that would be able to test him and had more knowledge of EB, if it was even EB. We said OK, but I wanted to go with him. My doctor said he would try to get me admitted into the other hospital, and if not, he would discharge me that day so I could go be with my baby. The Nurse brought him down to our room right before the ambulance took him away to the other hospital. Not long after that I was packed up and in my car driving to get there as soon as possible; I did not want to be away from him for one minute longer than I had to. This all happened less than 12 hours after giving birth to him, so I was still in a lot of pain and it was not easy for me to be rushing around. I was lucky to be able to be admitted into the hospital where they brought him, and as we arrived they put me in a wheel chair and brought me to my room, and then to my son.

Jonathan was once again in an incubator in the new Hospital and we still had no definite answers. Finally a dermatologist came in to speak with us; he thought that if he did have EB it was mild but had to do a biopsy to confirm the diagnosis and type. The dermatologist asked if I had any questions, and the only one I had was when I could hold my baby, and he told me that I could as soon as he finished the biopsy.

It was such a relief to finally have Jonathan in my arms. As I looked at him he smiled and I just felt at that point we would be okay no matter what lied ahead.

When the biopsy report came back, to all of our surprise, not only did he have EB but the Recessive Dystrophic form, which is one of the most severe types. Our hearts sank again as we were told all that could happen in our son's life. You go through a lot of emotions when you have a child with something wrong, and I think I went through them all. I kept wondering what I did in my pregnancy to cause this, even though the doctors told me it was nothing I did, I just couldn't help blame myself. The one thing that helped was how beautiful and content he was, considering everything. He only cried when doing his dressing, otherwise he was such a quiet and good baby.

We had to go through almost a week of being shown how to care for him to learn it well; learning to bandage a small baby is not easy. It took about four people to be able to hold him still and bandage him. Once we felt comfortable with caring for him we were able to take him home; I was excited yet nervous too. Would I be able to care for him properly? Would I do everything I needed to keep him alive? Most of all, how would I know what was normal baby things or his disorder?

The first year was difficult. Learning to just be a mom and learning to be a nurse all at once, it is a lot to take on for anyone.

Jonathan is now 8 years old. It has been a long 8 years but rewarding too. He was mild at birth but has progressed to be definitely RDEB. He has a lot of sores and blisters and scaring all over his body. As he gets older he is getting worse, but he is starting to help with his care making it a little bit easier. It is and will always be very difficult to care for him, but it has been very rewarding too. He has shown us how to enjoy the little things in life and not take things for granted.

My life has been dedicated to my children and always will be. They are everything to me. There are days that are great and I can't stop smiling but there are many days that all I want to do is cry. It is hard as a parent not to think ahead to the future. Most parents think about the day their children graduate from high school and get married. Having a child with EB makes you enjoy one day at a time, because you never know if you will see them graduate or get married. To all moms and dads, enjoy every minute of everyday like there will be no tomorrow. As an EB parent you have to worry if there will be a tomorrow.

~

Journey of Love

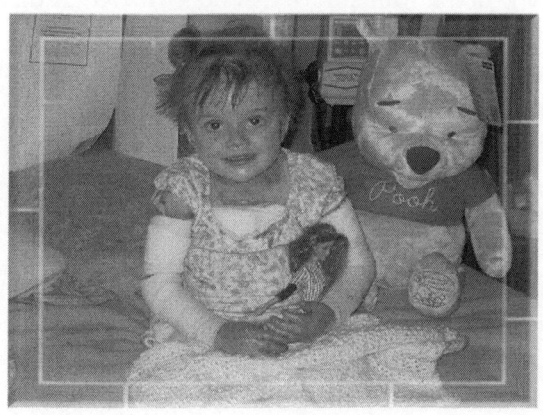

By Helen F.
helow143@optonline.net
ourgrace.org
New York, USA

Helen F. is Grandma (Me-Ma) to Grace P, who has RDEB. Grace is five and has six cousins free of EB. Helen is also an RN and until the birth of Grace had never heard of this disease. Her story tells of the impact of EB on her family and the compassionate love this tragic disease has sparked.

Good Friday 2002 was the beginning of a journey of love. Our Grace was born with no skin on her right foot, rushed to another hospital's NICU, leaving a path of confusion, pain and fear. Her mom and dad had dreamed of this birth, anticipating the joy and snuggle of their precious gift. Instead of having the time to cherish these special moments, Dad jumped in his car and followed his daughter in the ambulance, his mind in a fog, while mom lay in the hospital bed, anxious to sign her own release. "Not to worry," the doctors said. It was either Scalded Skin Disease or Epidermolysis Bullosa. They were 99.9% sure it was the former and that is cured by a course of antibiotics. Within 24 hours when the IV site was changed and Grace's skin came off at the same time, we all knew. Then we began a crash course in the nature of this dreadful disease that had a hold on our princess.

Grace's mom and dad became her greatest advocates, learning new terminologies, dressing changes, dealing with home care and case workers. No time to relish the moment, mom and dad rushed to get sheepskin and cover a car seat, buy special diapers and extra soft blankets. We learned about DEBRA and EBMRF and Recessive Dystrophic Epidermolysis Bullosa. We spoke with representatives of National Rehab and Mölnlycke. In the midst of this, Grace's parents dealt with grief and so did the entire family. No one sat with us and allowed us to name our pain. No one shared about this new path that was beginning with a child that had special needs. No one really allowed us to cry and discuss our fears as parents, grandparents, aunts and uncles.

We never heard of this disease and to compound the challenge, neither did most of the professional medical staff that surrounded us. "Be careful lifting her", "Always wear gloves and gowns and masks", "You can do this", "God doesn't give you anything you can't handle", and "God chose you to be Grace's parents"….these were the hackneyed phrases that well meaning people shared. However, when the tears came, most people were uncomfortable, they had no words. If they only knew we just needed to cry and that their presence would be enough. We were grieving for what could not be for our precious Grace, and we were angry. We were angry at everything and everyone and we needed to safely vent but there was no time and no compassionate shoulder. Our grief was building up and pushed aside because of the crises of the situation. How do we handle our feelings and care for our darling? What will Grace's future hold? What do they mean by life threatening? It hurts so much to see a little one you love in so much pain. We are thankful that now there is a family advocate program so no other families have to bear this alone.

Grace was loved before she was born and is loved now and will be forever. Because of a quirk in genetics, she suffers daily. Yes, there is a grief because our Princess cannot do what others can and we can't change that. She is not a victim nor was her birth a sad experience. It was just very different than expected and whenever that happens there is grief. As a family, we have learned to care for Grace. Slowly, her parents and family learned skills needed for Grace's well-being. It is a family illness since its touches us all. We have learned to share her story in the hopes that she can help other families. We have learned to advocate for awareness and a cure. We have learned to ask for help from friends and professional expertise. We have learned to beg and raise funds. We have learned to share feelings, cry together and have hope in the midst of desolation and we have learned to pray. Most of all, we have learned to enjoy the moments, the little smiles, belly laughs and the tickle nose games and we have learned to truly love butterflies.

Whenever someone stares or asks a question, we give them a little card with Grace's picture and a small explanation about EB. We pass out magnets, bracelets and newsletters and we have a website. Our Christmas letters are filled with requests for donations and prayers. This is our way of life. EB is not some distant orphan disease. It is in the face of our Grace and her friends, John Hudson, Robbie, Garrett, Brian and the many more who suffer until we get a cure.

We have been privileged to witness miracles happen because of our Grace. People have gathered to help, to pray, to build, to donate, to sing, to dance, to make us laugh and to just listen to our pain. This is the gift of EB. It touches souls and changes hearts. These innocent children are slowly teaching the world compassion, one heart at a time. Their little eyes tell of sadness and hope. Hope of a cure... hope for a magic potion for itch and hope that all will someday understand the devastating effects of this disease and overcome it forever. We share this prayer with all in the hopes of a cure.

Weaver of Dreams

Weaver of Dreams, to you we pray
Weave us a dream of a pain free day.
A Dream of skin that is smooth and clear
Of all the blisters and scars we fear.

Weave us a dream of riding a bike,
Even a dream of taking a hike.
Weave us a dream of jumping up high
A dream of never wanting to cry.

Weaver of dreams with magic thread
Please give us hope for what is ahead.
Weaver of dreams, this we beg,
A cure for this illness we so dread.

Weaver of dreams we are asking you,
To make all aware of this journey we do

Weaver of dreams heal our hurts
So when we awake we won't be worse.

Weaver of dreams be by our side,
To give us the courage to continue the ride.
Weaver of Dreams with magic thread
Touch all the people with what you have said.

Nothing is impossible through our God
Bless them all for working so hard.
Amen

Helen Farley
(Grace's Me-Ma)

~

Courage of the Heart

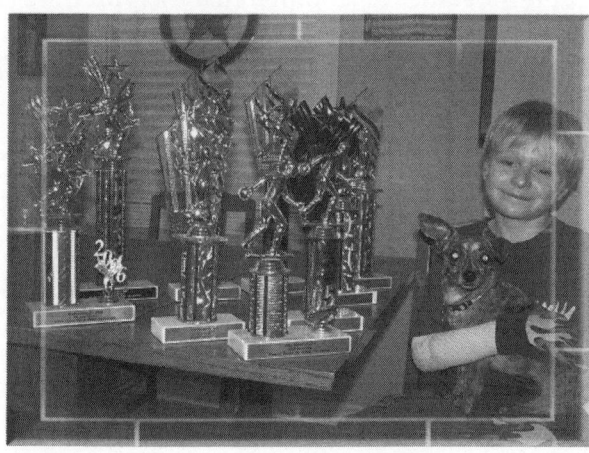

By Karen W.
kwalthall@verizon.net
Texas, USA

Karen W. was a 4th-grade teacher in Crosby, Texas when she taught Weston Z. She would like to share her story about watching "courage in action" each and every day as Weston attended her class.

Courage, raw courage. That's what I saw every single day as Weston entered the doors of my classroom. Here was an extremely intelligent, sweet, funny, articulate 4th-grader, trapped in a body that hurt constantly, would not allow him to run and play, and limited every single aspect of what we consider a "normal" life. However, it never limited Weston.

Weston refused to bow down to the disease. At times, the pain was so intense that he couldn't see, and his legs hurt so badly that he would lie down during our recess time to alleviate some of the stress on his wounds. Despite it all, he never EVER quit. In fact, when he was home he played with his animals, rode his 4-wheeler, and had a full life of love with his family. At school, he was a natural leader as the other children inherently recognized the strength of character that he carried within himself. He always had a calming presence in the room and entertained everyone with his jokes and stories.

I was the teacher, but I learned so much from this 10-year-old child. I learned that life is worth living to the fullest...whatever the cost.
I learned that no movement is too minimal to appreciate and no joy is too little to enjoy.
I learned that courage could be taught to others - courage of the heart. Courage to face the pain that will ALWAYS lie ahead, yet face it with a resolute smile and inner strength of character.
I learned to passionately love the fire that ran within the soul of this dynamic young man.
I learned to treasure the time that Weston was the teacher and taught me how to live more fully with all the blessings I ignorantly enjoy.
I learned about courage that walks among us each and every day.

Thank you Weston for making such an impact in my life!

~

My Blisters - No Fun!

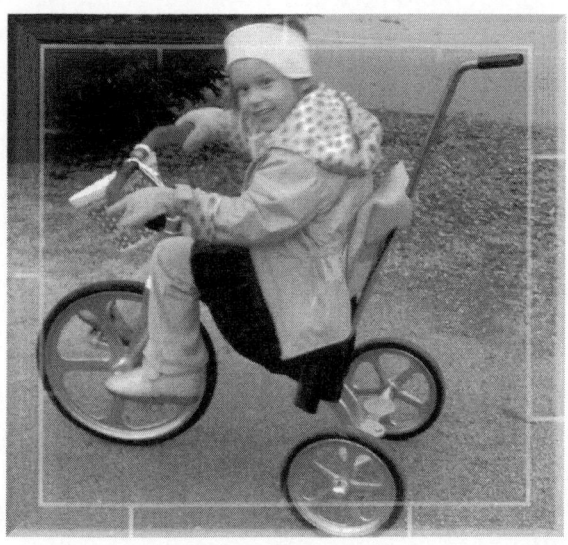

By *Christina M.*
camperminkey1@aol.com
California, USA

Christina M. is seven years old. She has EB Simplex, with the worst blisters on her hands and feet, although they occur in many other places. EB has gotten more challenging for her and she wanted to share her story. She lives with her mom, dad, 6 year old sister, and her 2 cats in Northern California. She wants to be a writer when she grows up.

Hi, my name is Christina. I am the only one in my family with EB.

I do not like to talk about my blisters. They make me sad. The worst part of my life is my blisters and other people have it too. It is no fun at all. It is very painful. People stare at me. People stare at me a lot. I stick my tongue out at them. People stare at me at stores, at parks - lots of places. Not at school- they know me there. I do not like it when people look at me funny or ask me what is wrong with me or did I fall down. They ask me if I ate strawberry jam, if I have blisters on my face. They ask stupid questions. I do not like it!! I do not like it all.

When I was in pre-school one boy said my blisters looked like poo.

That hurt my feelings really bad. That was a bad thing to say to me. God told me that I should not listen to him. I never forgot that.

Water is good for me so I swim a lot. I like to swim. I am taking swimming lessons. One time when I went to Tennessee they would not let me use the pool because they saw my blisters. I was really upset because I wanted to swim in the pool on my vacation. It was really hot out. It was 95 degrees. My mom was mad. She bought us a little pool to swim in at our aunt's house. It was not the same as a big pool. I like to go way under and swim in the deep end.

Sometime I cannot walk. I have a wheelchair. I had to get a new wheelchair and I miss my old one. My new one will have light up wheels but I still liked my old one. I have a tricycle that was made for me. It is easy to pedal. I use it at school. I ride really fast. I use it all day even at recess.

My feet get blisters really, really easy if I walk a lot. Sometimes a lot is just walking a little bit. Sometimes I ride on my dad's neck- that part is fun. I like to ride on my dad's neck. Sometimes he picks me up and it can hurt if he touches the places where the blisters are. I get blisters under my arms.

I feel different from other people. That does not feel good either. Let me tell you why- because people look at me different than their friends.

My best friend is my sister. She and I have the same room and lots of the same toys. She is not the same as me. She does not have blisters like me. She can do things I cannot do. She can jump and run really fast. She is going to take ice skating lessons this summer. I cannot do that.

I have to put a needle in my blisters. My mom used to do it all for me. Now I am seven and I try to do it myself too. I do not like it at all. Needles hurt. I have to drain the blisters- I use a lot of cottons. I put the needle in the puffy part and the fluid comes out. I have to put antibiotic cream on. It is really gooey. I have to cut my skin on my feet after a bath. It takes a long time. The skin is really loose and dangly. When I go swimming I wear socks so no one will see the skin on my feet. I put a towel over me at the pool when I get out of the water. I do not wear bandages a lot. Bandages make me get more blisters.

I wear special shoes. I use to only wear slippers. I wear crocs shoes now- I even have some with pink diamonds on them. People always say they like my shoes. I have to have my hair short or I get blisters on my neck. My sister has her hair long.

Sometimes I have to take medicine-it is really yucky too. Bleah! Bleah!! I wake up in the night and my feet really hurt. It hurts a lot. I have to get up and take medicine with my mom. It is no fun to get up in the night. My cat OB sleeps with me and my cat Leah sleeps with my mom and dad.

My family had an EB party at my house. I liked it very much because all our friends came. We put butterflies all over the house. It was really pretty. Did you know butterfly wings are like EB skin?

There is this person that had two EB children and they died- that is how bad EB is. Mommy tried to get lots of money to give to the doctors who are trying to cure EB. People came that did not know about EB and we told them all about it. We showed them pictures of lots of EB kids. People do not know that kids die of EB.

Thank you for listening to my story. Blisters are no fun!!!

~

Living with Epidermolysis Bullosa

Too Young To Die

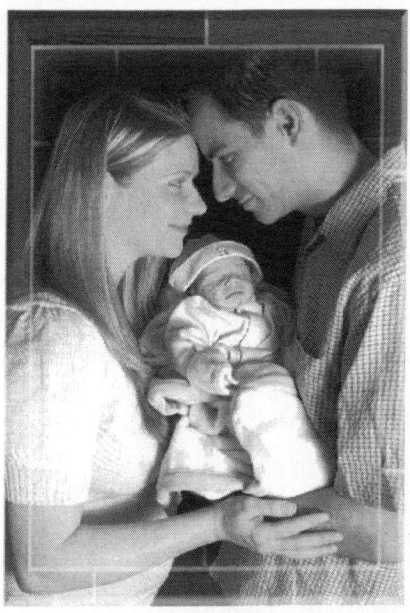

By *Amber O.*
XoSoulfuLxEyeSoX@aol.com
California, USA

Amber O. Is the mother of Zachary who was born with the Junctional Herlitz form of EB. Due to this form Zachary passed away at 3 and half weeks old. Their family resides in California, USA. Zachary was the first child born with EB in their entire family so naturally this came as a shock. This is their story and how they learned what EB was and learning to deal with it. They also had to learn to let go of their precious baby boy.

I am writing this for the one who can't, my son. While I was pregnant everything was fine, I was completely healthy and everything seemed perfect. Zachary was born early Sunday morning at 12:24 a.m. naturally without any complications. After 13 hours of labor, we thought our wait was finally over, until the awful truth was about to hit us.

Right after birth they let me hold Zachary for a very brief time (about 5 minutes) and then they rushed him out of the room. They wouldn't disclose exactly why they had to take him so suddenly, but they needed to talk to my husband in private and took him to go see Zachary in the nursery. Finally they came back and informed me of the situation; they said he was born with abnormally long fingernails and his skin was missing around his thumb. Quickly the pediatrician was called in and thankfully she had heard of EB before, so she knew right away what he had.

The Doctors decided that it would be best to call in a helicopter to transport him to a specialist in San Diego, as they thought an ambulance ride might be a little too long and traumatic to Zachary. Soon the helicopter crew arrived to pick our baby up, and just as quickly air lifted him down to Rady's Children Hospital in San Diego.

I was quickly discharged from the hospital seeing as I had no complications at all and would be fine as long as I took it easy. We then left the hospital and drove straight down to Rady's with my husband's mother and grandmother. By the time we got there it was now 5 a.m. Sunday morning; he was in an incubator with an IV in his foot.

The Nurses told us we were not allowed to hold our baby nor even just touch him. We continued to stay in San Diego over the next couple of days, and came in every single day to see our little boy suffer and we couldn't even hold his hand; we just sat there and watched him and talked to him through the incubator to tell him that mommy & daddy were there and that we loved him.

Each day we came back we saw our precious baby get more and more blisters all over his body. He went through dressing changes twice a day. All the nurses in the hospital said they had fallen in love with our precious little boy and just thought he was the most adorable boy they had ever seen.

The Doctors informed us that in order to take Zachary home we would have to learn how to perform the dressing changes; we had to learn how to pop his blisters and cover his whole body with Aquaphor and Mepitel and bandage him up.

By two weeks of age they felt we had a handle on how to complete the dressing changes and allowed Zachary to go home. The car ride home was extremely uncomfortable, as he had to be confined to a car seat. We had a rough first night home with him since he was more used to being up all-night and sleeping through the day. Everything was harder since we had nothing close to ready for him at home yet, except for his bassinet and baby things.

After having him home for two days he got sick again. With a fever of 103 we called his pediatrician and she told us to take him back to Rady's immediately, so once again we had to let go of our sweet little baby. By this time they had received the results from his biopsy and informed us with the heart breaking news. Zachary had Junctional Herlitz Epidermolysis Bullosa, and babies born with this type rarely live to see their first birthday, they also told us that Zachary didn't look like he could handle much more and that his little body was slowly giving up. By this point he was no longer eating which was a struggle from the beginning. Weighing 5 lbs. 8 oz. at birth, he had dropped to an even 5 lbs., so we did what any parents would: we chose to take our precious baby home to pass away surrounded by his loving parents and family.

The day we decided this, we opted to stay overnight in a hotel so we could pick him up first thing the next day. The following morning we took him home and spent as much time with our baby as we could. Once again we had to deal with the battle of securing him in his car seat and driving him all the way home from the hospital; luckily he just slept the entire ride home.

My husband and I had decided to use hospice care to help him pass in the most comfortable way possible. In order to hold him we had to give him morphine every four hours. Once we gave him his morphine we would just sit and cuddle him.

On his last night here, grandma and family stayed up all night with Zachary to watch over him and spend time with the last precious moments they had left with him. Two days later Zachary passed away in his daddy's arms while I held his hand. Zachary died from heart failure due to this disease.

By the time he passed away 80% of his body was an open wound. He died at 3 weeks and 5 days old; two days shy of being 1 month old. His grandparents from daddy's side unfortunately weren't able to make it in time before he passed but they were happy that they could be there for his funeral.

Zachary's funeral was beautiful and everything went perfect, especially the 21 doves that we released for him.

I wanted to tell Zachary's story because he is no longer here with us to tell it. He taught us such a huge lesson, that tomorrow is not promised to anyone and to cherish each moment you have with your loved ones. Zachary will forever be loved and missed by his Mommy & Daddy. We love you sweet baby boy!

~

Living with Epidermolysis Bullosa

Angel Sent From Heaven

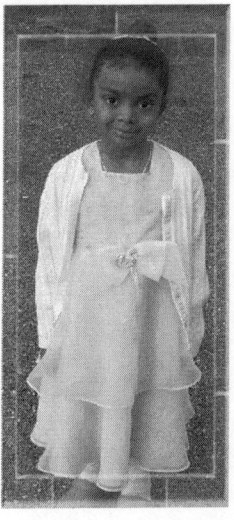

By Greg G.
melissag77@yahoo.com
Pennsylvania, USA

Greg G. is the father of McKenzie, a six year old little girl with Recessive Dystrophic EB. We live in Pennsylvania and our story tells about our little girl who was adopted with EB.

Everyone has heard the phase of new beginnings; well this is a true new beginning story. Both Missy and I have children to previous marriages. You have maybe heard of yours, mine, and ours. Well we had been missing the (our) part of the family.

We worked on conceiving naturally, In-vitro Fertilization, and the whole process of Missy taking shots. This was a very emotional time for us, we finally had some positive results, and found out we were finally pregnant. We had thought things had been going in the right direction but we had gone for a normal check up during the pregnancy at 5 months along, and we received devastating news: the baby had no heartbeat. Therefore, we were back to square one again.

We had discussed our options at this point, as to what we could do to fill this void in our life. We decided that we could help give a child a new beginning and give ourselves a new beginning by adoption. This truly was the start of a new beginning and firsts. The first time either one had even thought about adoption, this was very scary just due to the fact that we didn't even know where to begin, what the costs would be, if we could even afford it.

We made an appointment with a local adoption agency searching for answers and we found them, not all of them, but enough to know that this is truly what we wanted to do.

We will never forget the day that we received a phone call from the agency, who told us that they had a one-day old baby girl and asked us if we wanted to take her. They also told us that she had some skin problem.

We packed our bags and off we went to the hospital about four hours away from our home to find this precious miracle of life. There is no way on earth we could have walked away from this beautiful girl; I will never forget what my first words were: "She has a home, and it is with us no matter what skin problem she has."

The most wonderful gift that the good Lord has given us is this beautiful little girl. Her name is McKenzie. She has been diagnosed with Recessive Dystrophic EB. She spent the first fourteen days of her life in the pediatric intensive care unit due to the trauma from her birth.

McKenzie was born with no skin on her right leg from the knee to her little toes and her little fingers had been blistered along with several blisters on her face and various parts of her body. This was another one of those firsts; we never heard of the skin disorder nor did either one of us have any medical background to give her the attention medically. We did know one thing; that is, she would never lack TLC.

McKenzie was 1 year old on March 2nd, 2002, and she still had her right leg wrapped since birth and we changed her dressings daily. She was still getting blisters almost every day, but we stayed right after them, popping even the smallest of them to keep from filling up and getting bigger.

Our little girl is a real trooper; she will sit there and watch you take care of her sores with little to no resistance. She is doing very good, and is getting to the point of knowing what some of her restrictions are and she will avoid actions that she feels unsafe or she may get hurt. We helped her through the toddler stages with crawling and the beginning stages of walking with kneepads; they have been a blessing.

When she was little, McKenzie was enrolled in a day care center at a local church. We have worked with the employees at the center on what to look for, how to care for her; they were so wonderful to her. McKenzie would play on the mat and crawling around interacting with the other kids. McKenzie just loved it there with her new friends and especially Miss Marsha.

McKenzie sees a dermatologist regularly and her Dr. is very amazed with her progress, she is in the 90 to 95 percentile for her age group. We have learned through all of this that there is no magical treatment or care. It has been trial and error and again lots of TLC. We have found that in the summer months that any new or open wounds that are hard to heal areas, our swimming pool with the pool chemicals has been very helpful. The chemical appears to speed the healing by helping to dry out the affected areas. On the other hand, when her wounds are drying we apply vitamin E oils and various other moisturizing ointments to keep her from drying too fast and eliminate the chapping and cracking of her skin. We have also recently purchased a spa for McKenzie for the winter months, this works maybe even better for her. The water motion from the jets will help lift the old crusty skin to the point that it sheds by itself pain free. It has been great skin therapy for her.

We would like to thank all the wonderful people that we have met through our learning experience. It is nice to know that with everything that is going on in our society today, that we have so many kind and considerate people that we can reach out to.

We went to our first EB conference in Philadelphia in 2002. The conference was so educational and we learned so much from it, I would encourage that if you have not attended a conference that you would do so, not only for your own education, but I think it is good for the children to know that they are not alone in this. The conference was a large group of very kind and considerate people that all have something in common; the fight against EB. I strongly urge the support of the Debra foundation; they are doing so much good for this fight and we all need to keep the fight alive.

~

Living with Epidermolysis Bullosa

Our Story

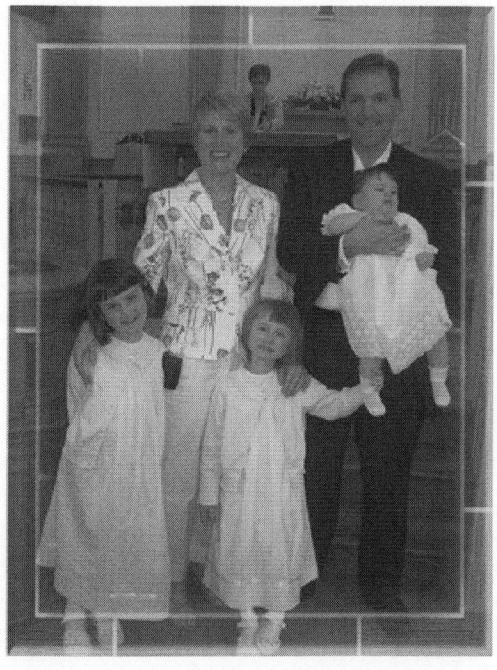

By Anna D.
California, USA

Anna is the mother of Anna, who has EB Simplex. This is her story.

It is May 21st, 2007, and today I went to visit my daughter, Anna's kindergarten teacher. I wanted to talk with her about Anna's progress and how I could best prepare my daughter for a full day of school next year when she starts first grade. For a moment, I thought I would cry. In the back of my head I was thinking, "What about the tough days?" Like the days when she tries to ride her bike to keep up with her sister and her bottom ends up red and blistered. Or the times when a simple gleeful skip can end up in bloody knees and hands and screams and tears. Then I am drawn back into the conversation again, "I know you have been through a lot with Anna, Mrs. Dittman, but you should know in many, many ways she is like most children." "Ok, I say, and fight back the tears, let's make a game plan for next year."

My name is Wendy and together with my husband, Todd we have 3 beautiful girls. Anna is our middle child and she was born in April of 2001. You always remember life before EB and then there is life after. I was one of those Moms who had a very easy first child and therefore, I probably thought I knew more than I really did. Suddenly, Anna was born and I (we) felt so vulnerable. Why was our baby missing skin on her wrists and ankles and why were her cries so "shrill"? The pain was evident and the shock for us was even more so.

"What is Epidermolysis Bullosa?" I asked the Chief of Neonatology at Ohio State University hospital who gently held my hand and tried to explain. As Anna was whisked away in an ambulance to Columbus Children's Hospital, I lay sobbing in my bed. Even though I am an insulin dependent diabetic, I begged my doctor to let me go so I could be with my baby.

Day after day was a blur and for the first time in our marriage, I saw my husband sob and sob. The blistering worsened and we feared our baby would never come home. By day 10 in the NICU, Anna's condition was so severe; she needed to be transferred to the Burn Unit. She would spend several days covered in bandages with blistering wounds over 90% of her body.

I remember begging God to save her and then as I held my little one as the nurses administered her morphine dose so she could withstand the pain of her bandage change, I just prayed "Thy will be done." How could I pray to keep her if she would live a life of such awful pain??? I had to rely on my faith as a compass and I just surrendered to having any answers or understanding of why something so awful could occur to a child - especially my own.

As more days passed, we finally saw a glimmer of hope. The Friday before Mother's Day in 2001, I walked through those hospital doors with my baby out into the beautiful spring day - a day no words can describe except to say, "one of great hope". That day was not without trepidation though. Boy was I worried.... How I would do it all...feeding tube, bandage changes that took 3 hours alone, special high calorie formula mixes, and prescriptions that I couldn't even hold in one hand. All that and a 20 month old at home, waiting for me. I begged God again "Please help Anna and help me too!"

From the tiny age of 2 months, we started with Occupational Therapy and Anna saw many specialists: There was G/I, surgery, and dermatology. You name it. We were either there or trying to get there.

I learned a valuable lesson. No one was going to have a "magical cure" for my daughter, but I could garner bits of wisdom from each person who helped my child and I just needed to keep plugging along.

Many of those days in her first year of life were a blur, but the role I now gained besides that of Mom was "advocate". That was a new role for me, but eventually one I became well suited. Having a child with EB can do many things to you as a parent. Anna's gift to me in all her suffering was to make me stronger and more courageous than I had ever been. How could I be anything but that for her? She deserves the best life my husband and I can provide for her.

So here I am today...crossing another milestone with my daughter and being so thankful for the opportunity to do it! First grade! I can't believe it. My precious Anna is my gift, but I also believe, a special gift to the world. Her life is a reminder of grace in suffering. She is the first to say: "I love you" the first to say: "I'm sorry" and guess what she wants to be when she grows up? A nurse! I know she'll be the most compassionate one out there.

The world needs more compassion - don't you think?

~

Living with Epidermolysis Bullosa

Our Angel Zachary

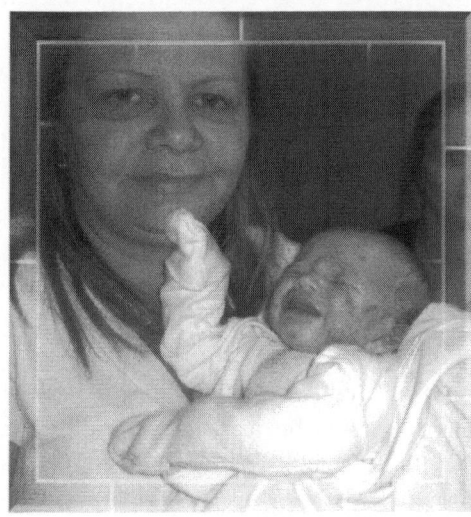

By Tammy H.
blueeyeslynn64@yahoo.com
California, USA

Tammy H. is Zachary's grandmother and in this tale she tells of her story of love and loss of her little grandson from Junctional Epidermolysis Bullosa.

Zachary Hayden was born on February 25th, 2007 to Amber and Chris. As soon as he was born the doctors noticed something wrong, he was soon sent to a NIC unit in San Diego, California. This was Amber and Chris' first child. They were two young parents and as they waited for the tests results from Stanford they prayed.

When the test came back they stated that Zachary had EB, the most severe case, Junctional Herlitz, the doctors called us all together for a meeting, Grandpa, Amber, Chris, auntie and myself. At the meeting they told us he did not have long to live and wanted to know what we wanted to do. We could keep him in the hospital or take him home and love and hold him while we could; his mommy did not want to see Zachary in any more pain, he was suffering.

I will never forget little Zachary or what I experienced with his life and death, Amber got to bring him home on her birthday March 21st, and little Zachary passed away on March 23rd so we only got 3 days with him, and in those 3 days we had a family photo with Amber, Chris and Zachary, taken also was one with grandma and grandpa. We loved him so much; I even took time off from work to help take care of little Zachary.

Let me tell you what that little angel went through: I had to feed him with a dropper because he could no longer eat from the sores in his throat, changing his little diapers was so painful for him. He passed away in his mommy and daddy's arms. I will never forget it, we prayed him into heaven and my daughter and son-in-law were so amazing, so strong, they saw the pain in their little angel and were willing to let him go instead of him going through any more pain.

I rocked Zachary all night and sang Jesus loves you, this I know and other songs, God knew what he was doing, he showed his grace when he came to our home on march 23, 2007 at 10:20 am and took little Zachary Hayden home. Amber said she felt the presence of God there with us and she kept on telling me pray mom, pray mom, help pray him in to heaven, Jesus is here, and I feel him.

Chris and Amber kept telling little Zachary, as he took his last breaths: It's ok baby, go with Jesus, mommy and daddy won't be mad at you, we will see you again, rest angel rest.

We had him baptized the night he came home; our pastor came to the house, everyone had a little time with him. God knew what he was doing...

We all love and miss you little Zachary, but God had better plans for you he only takes the best.

Love, grandma Tammy, Mommy, Daddy, Grandpa and Great Grandma Peggy who loves him very much and will miss him, she will see him again in heaven.

~

Living with Epidermolysis Bullosa

I'll Take My Angel Home

(Grandpa Greg wrote this poem for him when he passed away, he read it at the funeral, he misses his grandson very much and loves him)

From the moment we laid our eyes on you
it filled our hearts with joy.
For nine long months we felt you grow
and we knew it was a boy.

We held you close for a moment
before you were taken away.
But our world began to slowly change
with what they returned to say.

Our baby had a condition
both unique and oh so rare
That all at once our world looked bleak
and filled with much despair.

We began to do the only thing
which we have come to love.
We placed trust and all our worries
with our Lord above.

We asked him please take care of Zac
and heal him if you can.
But if you can't we'll understand
you had a different plan.

Through you our future is set
to us it is unknown.
We felt your presence on that day
and knew we weren't alone.

It was like you stood there silently
guiding us through this test.
And when that moment came to pass
we knew we had done our best.

Now Zac is in a better place
he sits beside your throne.

Because you came and said
I'LL TAKE MY ANGEL HOME.

I love you and I'll miss you Zachary, love grandpa

~

A Journey Into Motherhood

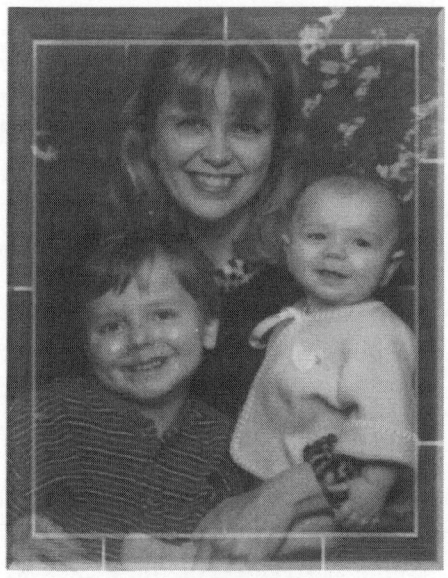

By Silvia C.
ebmomma@gmail.com
silviaskingdom.com
California, USA

Silvia C. Is the mother of Nicky, a 10 year old child with Recessive Dystrophic EB. Silvia lost her first baby at birth, Alex, most likely from EB, although it was not diagnosed at the time. She also has a healthy 3-year-old little boy, Connor. Her story highlights her losing Alex, her struggles taking care of Nicky, things she wishes she would have been told at birth and how her life has changed.

The story of my Journey into Motherhood and finding out the devastation that is EB didn't start when my son Nicholas was born in November 1996, but rather, 21 months earlier, on a sunny and warm day in Mesa, Arizona, when my first baby, Alex, was stillborn at full term. I will never say, however, that March 1st, 1995 was the worst day of my life, it was, after all, the one and only day in my life that I saw and got to hold my precious baby, one I will hold in my heart forever.

Alex was my first baby, my now ex-husband and I were extremely excited about this baby because we had waited several years to start a family. I remember vividly, as if it was yesterday, that feeling of 'something is wrong' when I woke up on Monday, February 27th, which happened to be the day after I was due. I called the Doctor and I went in with my mom to check things out. I will never forget what the doctor said while she placed the Doppler on my stomach: "Common Kido, don't worry your mom!" I noticed that the Dr a hard time finding the heartbeat, she then asked the nurse to bring in the ultrasound machine; at that point we were all staring at a baby that wasn't moving, no heartbeat, no nothing. He had died. The doctor could not give me any answers; she said we would have to wait to see the baby before a reason could be determined.

The Doctor sent me home to talk to my husband, and to decide what to do; only thing, he was at work. So that's where I went. I remember waiting for him at the receptionist desk; I had no idea what I was going to say to break the news. He came down the corridor with a big, big smile on his face, he thought we came to visit him to go to lunch together, but his expression turned quickly once he saw my face. He was worried instantly. "What's wrong? Tell me what's wrong?" I rambled something to go outside with me and once there I told him that the doctors couldn't find the heartbeat, the baby was dead. "Why?? How?" Answers I didn't know, what they told me at the perinatal office is that at this late stage it was most likely a cord accident, but we would have to wait to find out for sure.

That was indeed what I consider the worse day of my life. I shed more tears that day than the previous ten years combined. Nick went home with me, and from there we called the doctor to schedule an induction. I would have to wait that whole day and that following night before I could go in. I was in labor for 18.5 hours, 3.5 of those pushing; it all seemed like such a cruel joke. When he was born the doctor told me that Alex had the cord around his neck, which made it obvious it was a cord accident, but she was not convinced since it wasn't really that tight. What I did notice is how Alex's skin was peeling off all over his body, it was literally coming off in sheets. The doctors thought nothing of it, they told me that it is 'normal', and that the first thing that 'goes' in a stillborn baby is the skin. While that is true, I am still to see a picture of a stillborn baby whose skin looked as bad as Alex's did, and I saw hundreds.

Living with Epidermolysis Bullosa

Somehow for those few hours I spent with Alex I couldn't cry. I was in such an elated state to finally see him, comparing features with ours, and I was so proud. I would have done anything to hear him cry, ANYTHING!! Tears would not come until later, and they were flowing like a river.

Six months later, in September, I found out I was pregnant again, and I had a hard time feeling hopeful. Thoughtful friends sent me flowers and that cheered me up a bit, but this pregnancy was not meant to be. At nearly 8 weeks along I miscarried.

It wasn't until April of the following year that I finally got the news I was pregnant again. The doctors tested me for everything and it seemed like this baby was going to be okay. My main fear for this pregnancy was going to full term. In my mind, if Alex would have been induced a week early, he would be alive today, so my rationale was to make sure this baby would be induced at 38 or 39 weeks at the latest. The Doctor was not happy at all about this, and he did not hesitate to let us know. He told us many times that it would be a very long labor because I was not dilated at all, and he was less than pleasant about the whole thing. He did not realize how stressed both Nick and I were about this baby making it, we wanted him to be born alive, and we knew that he was alive at that moment. We did not want to take any chances and risk his life just to arrive at 40 weeks.

Nicky was actually due December 12, 1996, but one late evening on the 24th of November I left for the hospital ready to be induced. Labor was induced and things started going real fast at first, the water broke almost right away and I was at 10cm in just a couple of hours, but then everything slowed down considerably, and it was then that they realized he was posterior presentation, or "facing up". Nicky was not descending in the birth canal; so all my pushing was worthless. They tried to turn me around like a salami for 5 hours to make the baby turn, but they only succeeded in making the baby's heartbeat fall, which scared both Nick and myself to death. Even as Nick and I were crying, the doctor would continuously tell us "I told you so; the baby was not ready to come out".

It was now 7 pm, I had been in labor for almost 20 hours, and I was no closer to have this baby vaginally than I was 20 hours earlier, even if I was dilated to 10. Thankfully the end of Dr. L's shift finally arrived. A nurse took care of me until the Doctor on call came in. I will never forget this new Dr., he was an angel that came to save the day, and I truly believe it. As he entered the room he made everyone at ease. Both my mother-in-law and my mom were in the room, both Italian, and Dr.

A. (also Italian) started conversing to them in Italian! This Doctor was immediately concerned about the baby and me, and immediately suggested a C-section. He told us that he had also lost a son much like we had lost Alex, and that he understood our worries and concerns completely. He talked to Nick like a father, reassuring him and helping him. He told us that he would do his best. His best he did indeed and Nicky came into this world at 11:42 pm.

Our baby seemed just fine at first, even if early; he was good sized, lungs going great, and as cute as a button. We did not know it at the time, but being born C-section, hence being induced early, was the very best way for Nicky to be born, and the best thing that could have happened to him. If he had been born vaginally they would have torn his skin off on his head and who knows where else. He was certainly spared a lot of pain. Unfortunately, many other EB babies were not spared this pain, I have heard of babies being born without skin on many places of their little bodies because of the friction of passing through the birth canal.

Soon after he was born they showed him to me and he was absolutely perfect, he looked a lot like his big brother, but he had a much smaller mouth, had a lot less hair, he was blonde instead of dark haired... and, most important of all, he was breathing!!! They took him to the nursery to run all the newborn tests, and everything "looked" normal at first except for his mouth. After they aspirated all the liquids from his mouth it started bleeding and losing its skin.

At 4 am they finally brought him to me to nurse, and this was the first and last time I ever remember thinking of him as a normal baby, even with his mouth problems. I was cradling his little sleeping body in my arms and I was in heaven. The only thing that ruined the moment was my tiredness, I could not keep my eyes open, even with all the adrenaline of seeing and holding my baby! I felt like such a terrible mother. I had gone 2 complete nights without any sleep, I was hungry, tired and I felt horrible. There were tubes attached to me all over the place, but I was at peace seeing my little Nicky sleeping. He refused to nurse, but who could blame him? That was the one and only time that they ever brought him to me.

At around 8 am the pediatrician came into my room to tell me that they had to put Nicky in NICU in an incubator because of the problem with his mouth. They thought it was a "Staph Infection", "Herpes" or some rare skin disorder called "Epidermolysis Bullosa". By then, in fact, he had started blistering all over the place. They told me that they had contacted a dermatologist and that he would have come there that same morning on his way to the Children's Hospital in Phoenix from his office in Tucson.

When the Doctor arrived it was around noon, he told me that he had seen Nicky and did some sort of test with the eraser from a pencil and he wrote down the name of the skin disorder. He mumbled something about us having a 25% chance of this reoccurring in another pregnancy and then he wanted my signature on a piece of paper to let them take a skin sample for a biopsy. I was in a fog, I was drugged, I couldn't get out of bed on my own, I would throw up everything I tried to eat, and I still had not had a few good hours of sleep, so my mind was not clear, this is all I remember of Dr. H's visit unfortunately, aside the fact that he was very interested in seeing pictures of Alex.

It became obvious now, since Alex had all that skin coming off, that he also had Epidermolysis Bullosa. One Dr. with EB experience told me that EB fetuses are more likely to be stillborn (and miscarried) than a healthy baby... although he couldn't tell me why. That possibly explains my miscarriage as well. Alex had a lot of skin missing and peeling, which is classic of an EB patient. We will never know for sure what exactly killed him, if it was a cord accident like we assumed at the time, or the EB. Of course, for us, it is extremely hard to think that Alex was healthy. It is perhaps better that we'll never know for sure.

The nurse took me down to NICU in a wheelchair and then left me. I was stunned to see that my baby had been put in isolation. They had to put an IV on the baby because he could not eat since his mouth was in such a poor shape, and he was attached to a heart monitor and other things. He was in an incubator to keep him warm, had no clothes on him aside some bandages and the diaper. They were keeping the tubes attached to his tiny body with gauze. They could not use tape. The tape had already damaged his tummy, and the hospital bracelets that they had put on his ankles had done some serious damage as well. When the nurse finally put him in my arms I held him for what I thought was an eternity, and I kept staring at those horrible blisters, I had never seen anything like it. On the right side of his head there were a lot of little red marks where the skin had torn off. The nurse told me he got those spots when I was trying to push him out, he kept banging his head onto my bone. The heart monitor they had put onto his head when his heartbeat had fallen caused the other spots on his head.

I went back to see him later on with my mom and my mother-in-law, and it was there that Nick called me in tears. Earlier he had come to see us, and I had given him the name of that strange skin disorder. Now he had had the time to research the Internet about it, and he was completely devastated. He told me that he would most likely die from this. The neonatologists comforted us a lot, and told us that EB is something that could be lived with. Another nurse told us that he had seen a newborn with EB before that did not survive, but that was in much worse shape than Nicky and that, unlike him, this baby's wounds never healed. We did not know what to think.

The following day I walked on my own to see Nicky in NICU and I spent lots of time with him. I got discharged the morning after, Thanksgiving Day. I really didn't think I was ready because I was still in a lot of pain, and I didn't like going home without Nicky. Some people told me that they did not know how I could bear going home without Nicky, but I told them that last time I went home without my baby, Alex was in the morgue, and this time it was a lot easier knowing he was simply in NICU.

I went to the hospital every day even if I had to be put into a wheelchair from the pain once I entered the hospital. Every day I would spend hours holding him, talking to him, rocking him, feeding him... I could have never imagined to love a child as completely as I loved Nicky... yet I was so devastated both that I did not get to enjoy Alex this much, and that Nicky was in this much pain.

Since I was pumping the milk for Nicky I could not take too much medication for the pain, but I felt Nicky needed the breast milk more than I needed the pain to go away. The neonatologists told me that they could not let me take him home until they figured out a way to make him eat on his own.

Using a little creativity, the nurses and the neonatologists were successful in making him eat from a bottle. He could not suck much because his mouth was so sore, so they used a "Haberman feeder" to squeeze the milk into his mouth. They used some lydocaine for his mouth so the bottle would not cause any pain if he were to suck. This worked so well that within a couple of days Nicky was off the IV.

Now they wanted me to learn how to medicate his wounds and care for him in every way, so the following Monday night I spent it at the hospital in a room. The nurse instructed me how to care for him and I stayed in a regular hospital room with Nicky and my mother-in-law for the entire night and the next morning. I will never forget one nurse's comment on "how well we were dealing with this". But after the experience with Alex, we were just happy we could hold a living baby, blisters or not.

The dermatologist came back the following morning; he talked to us for a while and managed to really depress us. Over and over again he did not want to give us any hope for his survival. He told us that we would be in week after week to treat infections, if not worse, and totally painted an extremely bleak picture for us. Afterwards he took us step by step on how to care for his wounds taking extreme care in doing so.

Thinking back, there is a lot to be said of all the wrong things that this Dr. did. For starters, when he came to see Nicky the very first time, (when he was only a few hours old), he never told any of the nurses to puncture the blisters or how is the proper care for these types of wounds. Because blisters usually should not be popped (on a normal person), the nurses did not touch them, but with EB it is of extreme importance to drain and tear these blisters otherwise they can grow and grow and became really big. Because he failed to tell us this, Nicky was in real bad shape. Both elbows and half of both arms were completely skinless, and so were his ankles, the top of one hand, several fingers, one of his knees, the big toe on his right foot, several spots on his legs, and his chest. This Dr. could have painted a less bleak picture for us too. Knowing what we know now, unless a child is born with a severe Junctional form, as long as he's taken care of properly, he can be OK! Sure, he will be limited and in a lot of pain, but he can live with this. Needless to say, my husband and I were not very happy with him, and things only got worse.

When we went back to see the Dermatologist at Phoenix Children's Hospital a couple of weeks later, he brought in a lady who had lost a son from Junctional EB a few months earlier to help us and teach us proper wound care. When this lady saw our son, she immediately knew he could not possibly have the same form of EB that her son had, and that he was going to be OK. She showed us photos of her son and we could definitely see a difference. Nicky looked so good in fact that the dermatologist told us that most likely had that one form or EB that goes away after the first birthday. Hard to believe this Doctor could tell us one moment Nicky would die, and the next that his EB would go away.

Nicky thrived at home. When we brought him back to the hospital to see his nurses on Christmas Eve, (he was 1 month old) they were in awe on how well he was doing, this was a few days before the results of the biopsy came back confirming that Nicky had EB and classifying it as "Recessive Dystrophic".

When we went back to see the dermatologist when Nicky was 4.5 months old he took a pair of scissors and literally cut Nicky's skin from the bottom of the toe that was fusing without any anesthetic. Nicky screamed for hours. Needless to say we never saw this Dr. again, Nick was furious. We are more knowledgeable about EB than he is, and to get this kind of care from someone who is supposed to be an expert... I rather go without, thank you!! The real experts were the Drs at the EB clinic at Stanford University in San Francisco.

We took Nicky to Stanford twice when he was little, once when Nicky was 8 months old, and once when he was 14 months old. The first time they classified him as having "mild" dystrophic, but the second time, because of all the problems of vomiting blood, they unfortunately had to "upgrade" his condition as "medium", which has since been upgraded again to "medium-severe". At Stanford we had the opportunity to meet other children with EB and some adults too. We were also given the hope for a cure, as the EBMRF (Epidermolysis Bullosa Medical Research Foundation) resides there, and we also got to meet Lynn Anderson, who is the president and founder. The Andersons have lost two children to Recessive Dystrophic EB, Chuck at 27 from skin cancer, and Christine at 14 from heart failure. Both children suffered deformities of the hands and feet, chronic anemia, malnutrition, and growth retardation. The people at Stanford were very helpful but nobody really knows how to deal with this disorder day by day better than people that actually live with it. Other parents met personally or through the Internet better answered questions dealing with everyday problems.

Life with Nicky and EB has not been easy, especially for him. At first we were transformed into nurses, and knowing nothing about medicine there was much to learn. The parent of an EB baby cannot wear clothes that have buttons or anything that might cause a blister if rubbed against, cannot wear jewelry, including watches, and the nails have to be extremely short. The baby itself cannot wear anything that has too many buttons, or is harsh (like jeans), it needs to be soft and easy to put on with a large hole for his head to pass through without needing to do any pulling. Everything has to be padded, from the stroller to the bed, from the swing to the playpen.

The first six weeks at home I was lucky to have my mom's help. I would sleep cradling Nicky, I was too afraid to let him sleep alone in his bassinet, even if it was just next to my bed, then, in the morning, I would give him to my mom so I could catch a few zzz.

Living with Epidermolysis Bullosa

I took advantage of it until she left, and then I went practically without any sleep for the following 2 months. Nick, who went to work, slept in the other bedroom for that time. Afterwards Nicky seemed to get the hang of sleeping, but even when he was 3.5 years old he still woke up at least twice a night, and only slept a total of about 7 hrs.; his afternoon nap could be between 1-4 hrs., there was no telling.

Until Nicky was 4 months old he had to wear mittens to protect his face from scratches, and then wore gloves that were made of Lycra and were elastic, so that the tips of his fingers could be free. One by one, I watched all his fingernails fall off, and taking care of his hands is a big job. His fingers have a tendency of contracting and webbing, and if this problem is not taken care of he will not have hands when he grows up.

Having the Dystrophic form of EB means also having the "disfiguring" kind. If an area gets too many blisters it will never regain its normal look, it will be reddish and squams). Disfiguring also means that his hands and feet can web and contract, and his mouth and esophagus are severely involved. Because of this he can only eat mushy or liquid foods, and needs to be drinking constantly to keep the moisture. He has thrown up blood every now and then from a popped blister in his throat. Because of this, he built scar tissue in his esophagus and has needed dilatations every few months to enlarge the passage of food. It got so severe we had to put a g-tube to supply to him enough nutrition. It is hard to brush his teeth, and his tongue always has blisters. The tongue has somewhat healed attached to the bottom of his mouth, so he has a lot less use of it as a normal person. He also has very little gum space, as the skin has fused there as well.

Nicky was 7 months old the first time I was able to give him a real bath (meaning... immerse him in water), and his baths do take a few hours because all his bandages need to be changed afterwards. He watched Barney or Blue's clues while mommy medicated and bandaged all his wounds, and then padded areas such as his knees, ankles, elbows, armpits, and chest etcetera. I never had any help, not even when he was a baby; I always had to do his bandage changes by myself. All of this is extremely time consuming, and thankfully, as time went by, Nicky has become more and more patient and cooperative.

Nicky was an extremely bright and careful little guy, he knew he could get hurt, so he took his time in learning skills that might hurt him. He practiced crawling for almost 4 months (from when he was about 8 months old) before he was actually able to do it. And he did it extremely slowly at first... and backwards!! He was 20 months old before he mustered up enough courage to walk on his own, but it wasn't until after his second birthday that he was able to truly walk on his own without help and without falling.

Taking care of Nicky per se improved dramatically from the time he turned about five years old, and while it's been easier in some ways, it was harder in others.

It's been easier because if he cried or got hurt he could now simply tell me where the owie was; before it was just a guessing game.

It's been easier because he would now sit still during bandage changes and even help me a little instead of screaming and kicking.

It's been easier because he could now entertain himself and I could talk to him and have a conversation while I bandaged him. The things he said were so cute! I loved this age.

However, things were harder too.

They were now harder because, with RD, he already had areas that wouldn't heal or would heal only to be open wounds again in a matter of a few days.

Harder because he could now tell me that he was in pain and where, so I knew he really was in pain.

Harder because now he knew he could not go out and run and play with the other kids because they would 'hurt him' (his words).

Things could improve though, and I knew they would eventually. I really hated, for example, when Nicky jerked away when I was trying to take off certain gauzes. If it was stuck or was a bit sticky he would actually hurt himself, while if he would have just stood still and I could take it off slowly, I wouldn't have hurt him at all.

I've always tried to have an open line of communication with Nicky ever since he could understand what I was saying. When he complained and cried in anticipation of a bandage change or a bath I would tell him: "Mamma does not want to do this either, but we *have* to do it so you don't get sick!" The last thing I wanted was for him to hate me or resent me for doing something I had no choice to do. I wanted him to understand and know that what has to be done needs to be accomplished without complaining. I didn't mind if he cried if he was in pain, but this "anticipation" screams were not acceptable to me. As much as I've hated doing bandage changes over the years I have never complained to him about them, and I always tried to make it a game for him, even though it was rough sometimes. Overall, however, things were easier. It's impossible to say if I was now just more 'used to it' and how it now was simply a way of life, while when he was a new baby, being not only new at parenting, but new in the nursing business, I was overwhelmed. I still was overwhelmed, but only because everything was on my shoulders. Nicky has always been my joy, and truly my reason for not going off the deep end at times. He has always been such a happy little kid, how can I feel depressed with such a cheerful little boy around?

His first hand surgery to undo the webbing and contracting on his right hand was performed just before his second birthday and it was an awful experience. The problem was not the surgery itself, but the recovery and the making sure that the fingers healed with no webbing and straight and keeping them that way. In November 1999 Nicky went through another hand surgery, this time on his left hand. The surgery itself was a little easier, but the recovery was a nightmare, and the hand did not heal right. In the summer 2002 we tried again to fix the left hand, and this time the surgery and recovery went very well. As I write this, in the summer of 2007, Nicky wants a few of his fingers 'done' and we're working on this.

My husband and I divorced in 1999 and life was hard for a while before I got re-married. Thankfully mommy did not have to work full time outside the home for too long. After one year and a half mommy was finally able to work from home. Nicky talks to daddy daily on the phone and they have a very close relationship. Mommy remarried and Nicky inherited a stepsister and her half brother aside from a loving step-dad.
In 2003 Nicky also got a little brother! He just loves his little 'pumpkin' as he calls him, and they are great friends, always playing video games together, or outside, or taking a bath together.

It goes without saying that I was scared to death during this new pregnancy. After a stillborn baby, a miscarriage, and a baby with EB, I felt like I was walking on needles for the entire nine months. The only reason I went ahead and tried to have a baby again was because this baby would have a different father; hence the chance of this baby having EB would be extremely small since both parents need to be carriers. Even though the chances of having another EB baby were next to none, I still worried. I was 39 years old and there were other concerns, such as Down syndrome for example. An Amnio was done, however, ruling everything out and we hoped for the best. On September 5th, Connor came into this world, healthy and happy! I still can't believe it as I watch him run around now, almost 4 years old.

Nicky is extremely bright and has finished on top of his class all the way from kindergarten through 5th grade. His teachers and aides have always been very impressed on how hard he works and how fast he learns. We are all very proud of him.

Health wise I wish I could say he's doing good or at least stay the same, but unfortunately that is not the truth. Nicky's health problems seem overwhelming at times. There are the endless bandage changes, the blood transfusions, the dental issues, hand surgery issues, throat issues, g-tube and nutrition issues, bowel issues... the ladder being the cause of much frustration, as family and friends cannot comprehend the condition and over and over again tell me I must be lazy or something... lazy? Do they really think I enjoy changing the diaper of a ten year old?

What has been the cause of most of the frustration and stress; however, were none of these things. It was the various Insurance Companies denying life sustaining/saving supplies, such as bandages to cover the wounds, or Pediasure/Nutren for his g-tube, denied my son to be seen and operated on by competent Doctors, and the constant, unending fight to make people understand that my son's condition really is as bad as I describe, and even on a good day, I couldn't exaggerate if I wanted to. How stressful is it for people to tell me that I am just trying to get pity from them... especially Insurance Companies, and their 'oh well, we're not going to cover it anyway' type of attitude. It all makes the stress and frustration turn into anger and that is when I have to sit down and just breathe.

Somehow, someway, I've kept my wits about me. Nicky is 10 years old as I write this, and while he's very bright and a joy, he cannot dress himself, feed himself, clean himself and will most likely never be able to. After his little brother was born I was left with the decision to get Nicky a power chair because I was in the predicament of not being able to go anywhere with both boys if I had to push a stroller and a wheelchair. While I had some friends who frowned on me for doing so, feeling that it would lead to Nicky becoming dependent on it, at the time I truly felt I had no choice other than growing another pair of hands! I never regretted that decision. Nicky has gained an extraordinary amount of independence from it and since he's not allowed to bring it into the house, he still needs to get around the house on his own two feet, albeit slowly. Because of the chair, he has a blast at school or at camp, being able to keep up with his peers and go anywhere (or almost!) they go. We wouldn't have it any other way.

I am not sure what the future will bring. It's hard for me to think about what lies ahead. Having the Recessive Dystrophic form of EB I know what's coming and I am always learning. My goal is to keep him as

Living with Epidermolysis Bullosa

healthy and happy as long as possible. If he lived to see a cure, that would be bonus! Perhaps Erma Bombeck, in her 'God chooses mom for a special need child' was right... as a mother of a special need child, we need to be happy, selfish, have a sense of self and independence. We need all of these things to be advocates for our children, to teach our children to live in a world that is not equipped for people that are different and don't fit into a certain mold... and stress and frustrations are, sadly, part of the game.

~

Poems

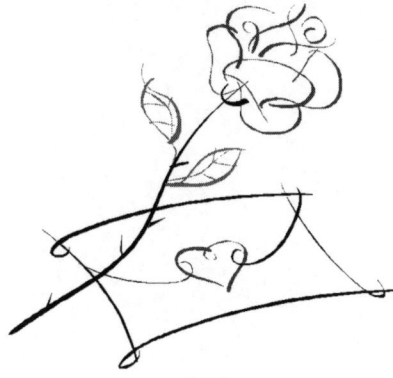

They may always wear bandages, please don't stare
Greet them with a smile that will fill the air
Look into their eyes and, what you'll see
Are Angels...and not the EB.

Written by Andrea Olinger

Living with Epidermolysis Bullosa

A Mother's Wish
(in memory of Garrett)

I gave birth to you, my precious angel
I thought everything would be fine
How was I to know
Your life would be shorter than mine?

You had lots of friends
Waiting at the gate
We now begin to see
This was your fate.

You ran to heaven
And couldn't wait to see
Your whole new world
That is EB Free.

You have no more blisters
You are in no more pain
But then again, life without you
Will never be the same.

To see you grow up
Was my biggest wish
What I wouldn't give
Just to feel your gentle kiss

Why God needed you now
We'll never know
What I wouldn't give to see you;
Only I will ever know

When I close my eyes I see you
You are never very far
Because in my heart
Always you are

~ Sara Denslaw, February 2005 ~

Baby Butterfly

The butterfly landed on our lives,
A precious and fragile gift.
Her beauty brightened every day,
But she was not meant to stay.

For then like all of those with wings
She longed to fly away.
She sought a place of perfect peace,
A home where pain would cease.

One day we'll be there with her
To enjoy God's paradise.
The time apart will disappear,
And forever we'll be near.

Goodbye, til then, our daughter.
Go on to the place you belong.
Dream big our baby butterfly.
Now spread your wings and fly.

~ Mandy Herreid ~

This poem was written for my daughter, Jordan. I wrote it for her funeral
program about five days before she went to heaven.

My Hero

My hero is not an actor or actress.
My hero is not an athlete.
My hero is not a great historian.
My hero is someone with incredible strength and courage.
My hero is someone who inspires many.
My hero is someone who endures pain daily, and still manages to go on and even
smile.
My hero is someone who to many may not seem beautiful, but to me is gorgeous.
My hero is someone who makes me laugh, makes me cry, and makes me proud every
minute of every day.

My hero is an EB baby, an EB child, and An EB Adult.

Dedicated and inspired by my son Jonathan

Love, Mommy (Brenda G.)

To Jessica

I never thought about
What special gift
I will get from God.
A little girl in my arms.

Never thought about
How special you
Are in my life.
You are the inspiration
Of my life who keeps
Me alive.

Every day
I see you struggling
In pain.
But through all
Your courage and smiles
You make me strong

Even when I feel too much
Pain down my heart
And feel my tears down
My eyes and heart.
I still thank God for the
Special gift you are.

You are my joy, life and
Whole world.
My prices who bought my life.

To Jessica From Mom

Resources

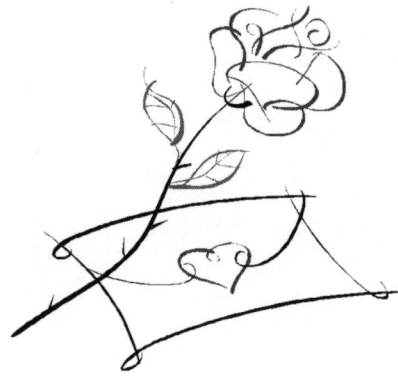

The following information is accurate as of June 2015

DebRA Organizations

DebRA of America, Inc.
75 Broad Street
Suite 300
New York, NY 10004

Phone: (212) 868-1573
Toll-Free: (855) CURE-4-EB
Fax: (212) 868-9296
Email: staff@debra.org

EB Nurse Educator, Geri Kelly, R.N.,BSN:
Phone: (866) 332-7276, (866) DEBRA-RN
Internet: http://www.debra.org
Email: nursegeri@debra.org

DebRA-United Kingdom
13 Wellington Business Park
Dukes Ride
Crowthorne
Berkshire
RG45 6LS

Tel: 01344 771961
Fax: 01344 762661
Email: debra@debra.org.uk
Internet: http://www.debra.org.uk
Internet: http://www.debra-international.org/

For a complete listing of all DebRA (Dystrophic Epidermolysis Bullosa Research Association) around the world, please visit this website:
http://www.debra-international.org/debra/national-eb-groups.html

Misc. EB Organizations/Centers/Websites

EB Medical Research Foundation
8909 W. Olympic Blvd. #222
Beverly Hills, CA. 90211
Telephone: 1-310-854-0957
Email: a.pett@bgent.com
Internet: http://www. ebkids.org

EB Research Partnership
132 East 43rd Street, Suite 432
New York, NY 10017
Email: info@ebresearch.org
Telephone: (212) 554-1467
Internet: http://www.ebresearch.org

Stanford EB Clinic
770 Welch Road, Suite 300
Palo Alto, CA 94304
Telephone: 1 (650) 725-9961
Telephone: 1 (650) 804-4820
Internet: http://dermatology.stanford.edu/gsdc/eb_clinic

Cincinnati Children's Hospital EB Center
3333 Burnet Avenue,
Cincinnati, Ohio 45229-3039
Telephone: 1-513-636-4200
Telephone: 1-800-344-2462
TTY: 513-636-4900
Internet: http://www.cincinnatichildrens.org

EB Info World
Internet: http://www.ebinfoworld.com

Summary Camps

CAMP WONDER

Internet: www.csdf.org
Telephone: 925-947-3825
Fax: 925-947-2158
Livermore, CA

CAMP HORIZON

Internet: www.aad.org
Millville, PA

CAMP DISCOVERY

Internet: www.campdiscovery.org
Telephone: 847-240-1737
Email: jmueller@aad.org

Thank you for reading!

Dear Reader,

I hope you enjoyed *Living with Epidermolysis Bullosa*. I took the initiative of compiling stories of families living with EB to give you a glimpse of what it's like to have walked in the shoes of a parent or patient who faced this condition. It was also my hope to give knowledge or a helping hand to other parents in similar situations, but my main intention was to raise awareness for this brutal disorder, called "The worst condition you never heard of". Without awareness there is no funding, without funding there is no research, and without research there is no cure. Please visit either the EBMRF (http://www.ebkids.org) or the EBRP (http://ebresearch.org) for more information on studies currently funded.

Finally, I need to ask a favor. If you were so inclined, I'd love a review of *Living with Epidermolysis Bullosa*. Loved it, hated it-I'd just enjoy your feedback. Reviews can be tough to come by these days, and you, the reader, have the power to make or break a book. If you have the time, here's the link to my author's page, along with all my books on Amazon: http://amzn.to/1InZdhY

Thank you so much for reading *Living with Epidermolysis Bullosa* and for spending time with us.

In gratitude,

Silvia Corradin

Printed in Great Britain
by Amazon.co.uk, Ltd.,
Marston Gate.